How to Cope Better When Someone You Love Has Cancer

Second Edition

WILLIAM PENZER, PH.D.

Esperance Press Inc.
150 South University Drive
Plantation, FL 33324
954 475 1371
cancerville.com

Second Edition *May 2013*

This book is available at special quantity discounts for bulk purchases, fundraising, educational, or institutional use.

Contact media@cancerville.com

ISBN-10: 098350170X

EAN-13: 9780983501701

Library of Congress Control Number: 2011932508

Printed in the United States of America

10 9 8 7 6 5 4 3 2 1

Better to light a candle than to curse the darkness.

–Confucius

If I can stop one heart from breaking,
I shall not live in vain:
If I can ease one life the aching,
Or cool one pain,
Or help one fainting robin
unto his nest again,
I shall not live in vain.

–Emily Dickinson

Of all the forces that make for a better world, none is so indispensable, none so powerful as hope. Without hope man is only half alive.

–Charles Sawyer

Dedication

My book is dedicated to all of the family, friends, and their loved ones who have dealt with cancer; all who are dealing with it now; and all who will have to deal with it in the future. I wish you safe passage and Godspeed.

It is also dedicated to the devoted researchers, physicians, and medical teams. It pays tribute to everyone working at cancer centers all over the world. This includes the receptionist at the front desk, the nurses, the directors of these centers, and everyone in between these important positions.

We are all joined together by a common bond of offering help and hope to those fighting cancer. Let us continue to work together to make this book, and all others on this topic, obsolete in the near future.

In the meantime, let us continue to extend a strong, warm, and caring hand of support wherever it is needed.

William Penzer, Ph.D.

Acknowledgements

I have been blessed to have had a solid team of support throughout my career, as far back as my first job as a psychologist for the IBM Corporation, my time as Assistant Director at The Institute for Human Development at Nova University in Ft. Lauderdale, throughout my almost twenty years as Director of the Center for Counseling Services, and throughout my years in private practice up to the present time. I thank you all for contributing to my life and my work in meaningful ways.

As for this book, the following deserve special recognition and thanks:

My wife and loving partner for more than fifty years, Ronnie, who not only coped well with my "obsession" for this book in the past year, but who also sat side-by-side with me and dutifully (and sometimes tearfully) sharpened her pencil for the first round of editing, which often took five or more revisions per chapter. Then, in her detailed and methodical manner, she spent over two hundred hours reading every word and comma aloud to me, helping me revise, revitalize, and finalize this book.

My special daughter, Jodi Mi, who provided us all with a role model of quiet strength as she faced cancer squarely, solidly, and successfully as she bravely led us through this difficult maze.

My son-in-law, Zev, who was and is a steady source of companionship, strength, and loving support for Jodi and our family.

My son Michael, whose sensitive side was challenged by Jodi's struggles, but who still brought much to the table of support including our fairy tale experience.

My son David and his wife, Lisa, for being there for our family and for David's ongoing encouragement for me to keep writing as he read the drafts of this manuscript. He is also helping with marketing and distributing this book.

My grandsons, Jarrett and Dillon, for making me happy and making me laugh whenever I see them. I am pleased to see they seem to have inherited my sense of humor.

My new friend Rob, who unwittingly lit the fuse of confidence as this book rattled around in my mind for five long years. He also worked tirelessly to contribute his edits to smooth and add to my words. His feedback woke me up to the fact that this book was not quite finished, when I was led to believe that it was.

Susan, who read the draft while battling cancer and provided excellent feedback and encouragement. She inspired the book, *How to Cope Better When You Have Cancer.*

Antje, a multi-cancer survivor, who read the Introduction and said, "You got it, keep writing!" She also created the beautiful glass sculpture shown at cancerville.com.

Linda, who demonstrated how someone can be truly and completely there for loved ones who have cancer.

My longtime friend and colleague Harvey, a psychologist, author, and publisher, whose wise and seasoned advice and encouragement guided me through this complex process.

Brad, who worked tirelessly into the night to keep my writings organized, graphically aligned, and together in ways my computer illiteracy would not allow me to do. He also did the illustrations at those late hours.

Jose who skillfully designed the cancerville.com website.

Babs, who designed the cover of this book.

Maria, who helped me by doing much research on a variety of related subjects.

Kerri, who arrived in the nick of time to do the final edits of this book.

Mimi, mother of a young survivor, who served as an extra pair of eyes and provided her feedback.

My therapist, Karen, who helped me clear my mind over the past three years so that I could confidently and coherently write this book

My friends and colleagues: Max, Neviana, Eileen, Joyce, Mimi, Shelly, Shelley Y., Randy, Erin, Shelley S., and Ellen. They all immediately believed I could do this and do it well. The bar they raised by their faith in me pushed me to overachieve.

All the unnamed people in South Florida who entrusted me with their minds all these years. Together we learned how minds work, why they sometimes don't work well, and most importantly, we learned how to help repair them. The courage and confidence they displayed in the face of adversity helped me to strengthen my resolve in my life and in Cancerville.

My heartfelt thanks and sincere gratitude goes out to all of you.

With love and much appreciation,

Bill

Table of Contents

Part III: Making the Land Your Own

Part IV: Tools That Help You Tend the Land

Part V: Putting Distance Between Yourself and the Land

Preface

As I began to write this book, I created a personal image of excellence. I wanted it to push me to write an exceptional book about a less than exceptional topic. The image I chose was symbolic of my goal. I was determined to write a clear and powerful book that would truly help people. I wanted to "knock it out of the park."

As a kid who grew up in the Bronx, New York, in the 1940s and 1950s, I was an avid baseball fan who spent a fair amount of time at Yankee Stadium. I therefore picked the following image to motivate me to write the very best book that I could.

It is the seventh game of the World Series, and the Yankees are playing their hearts out in their old stadium on Jerome Avenue. It is the bottom of the ninth inning, and we are down by three runs. There are two outs, and the count is three balls and two strikes. The bases are loaded, and I am at bat. I need to hit a home run—nothing less. That walk-off hit will give us the game and the series.

I want to hear their announcer of old, Mel Allen, screaming at the top of his lungs, saying, "There is a high fly ball to deep, deep center field. That ball is going, going, and it's gone. The Yankees win the championship. What a hit, what a game, what a series, what a win!"

That was the image I kept in mind while writing this book. I swung as hard as I could and aimed it right at you. I sincerely hope you will catch that ball and that my words will help you to stand tall during a difficult time. That is much more important than the outcome of a baseball game.

I want you and your loved one to win. That is really all I care about.

Introduction

I am sincerely sorry that you need to read this book. I wish you could be reading Danielle Steel, John Grisham, or any other book of your choice. I so wish that your life and your loved one's life were lighter, brighter, and free of suffering and worry. I hope you get back to that space soon. In the meantime, you have made a good choice. My words will help you through. They have helped many before you. They will help you too. I will walk you through this most difficult situation, while helping you hang tough and remain strong.

Most authors, I would imagine, want everyone to read their books. Oddly enough, I want no one to need to read this one. My sincere hope is that this book will become obsolete very soon. I want cancer to be a thing of the past and cancer centers to become empty ghost towns. That may not happen in my lifetime, but I am hoping it will happen. We are closer than ever before—we will get there! For now, I hope you will choose to read this book as a way to gain added strength and support at a difficult time.

Please know that I wrote this introduction in the same pained and screeching tone with which I viewed the world when my daughter was initially diagnosed with cancer. Yet I soon realized this angry and fearful approach was not the best way to deal with such a serious problem, and I learned how to adopt a more positive, comfortable, and comforting position.

As you continue to read this book, you will find that my voice and its tone and timbre soften, lighten, and seek out hopefulness and optimism in every nook and cranny. My only goal is to help you find those spaces sooner than I did, so you can rise more quickly to the challenge of having a loved one with cancer.

For some, my intro is a difficult read, but my book, I believe, is not.

Nothing—and I mean nothing—prepares a person for dealing with someone they love having cancer. On July 8, 2005, I knew that someday, if I lived long enough, I would write this book for you. At that time, living long didn't seem quite so important as it previously did or does now. On that torturous day, forever etched onto my brain like a permanent tattoo, I sat in the waiting room of Memorial Sloan-Kettering Cancer Center in New York City.

My wife and I were surrounded by other weary, bleary, and teary-eyed, seriously sad, and silent people. We were all ruminating about our collective fates and that of our loved ones. In our minds, as we each stared blankly into space like a room full of zombies, our loved ones were in serious trouble and we felt totally helpless.

So tilted was the windmill of my mind as it whirled and swirled frantically that I didn't know what to do or say or where to put all of the hyper-fueled energy racing through my mind and body. My wife and I struggled to find our way through this wasteland in order to stay sane, help our daughter, and survive the ordeal, as individuals and as a couple. I am pleased to say that we succeeded even though it took us a while.

Somehow, we stumbled and fumbled our way through, experiencing a wide range of overwhelming emotions. People who have a loved one dealing with cancer, people I have come to call "heart and soul givers" experience terrorizing fear, rage, confusion, and despair, not to mention a level of depression and anguish of unparalleled proportion. For most people, it is like no other challenge they have ever encountered.

On that day at Sloan-Kettering, I realized many things. I already knew from my work as a psychologist and psychotherapist that life wasn't always fair, but my experience helping others did not immediately prepare me for helping my family and myself. I was as lost as a tourist in a strange and foreign land, unable to get my bearings or even speak the language. There was no voice of support to hold me up. That is why I knew I would write this book someday.

To get through this difficult territory, you need a strong voice to lead the way. I am honored you are allowing me to be that voice for you. I take that responsibility very seriously. I will teach you how to provide that strength for yourself and your loved one. I have written the book I needed to read that day in the waiting room at Sloan-Kettering.

As we sat there quietly waiting for our daughter's procedure to begin, my mind was numb, as if frozen by an icy cold frost on a winter's morning in Montana. When the nurse called Jodi's name, signaling her turn, she, dressed in a gray hospital gown, stood up quickly and bravely. A single angry thought shot through my head in outraged indignation: "This cannot be my daughter's turn!"

As Jodi took the first step toward the operating room, elephant-sized tears began to fall down her cheeks as if she were a prisoner on her way to execution. Yet, in reality, she was an innocent victim of cancer. My frozen mind thawed and instantly overheated, as if I had been thrust headfirst into an oven. My heart skipped multiple beats; I was helpless to prevent the ensuing barbarism. Jodi had to walk these steps on her own.

At that very moment, I realized that cancer was not only a horrible and hated medical diagnosis, but it was a place as well. I knew then that my daughter, my wife, and I had entered what I came to call Cancerville.

Consider this book a guide to a place you really never wanted to visit. Like Jodi, your loved one was never given a choice—just a by-invitation-only command in the form of an X-ray, MRI, blood test, biopsy, or any combination of the above.

As our beautiful thirty-one-year-old daughter was led into the operating room for a mastectomy, we shakily made our way back to the waiting room. It was Jodi's boyfriend, Zev, whom we hardly knew; my wife, Ronnie; and myself. Jodi and Zev had been living together for less than six months. To his credit, Zev did not bolt. He is a very special man, as not all men stay the course. Over the years, since that day at Sloan-Kettering,

Ronnie and I have become very close to Zev and love him as our own. At the end of this book, I will tell you the very special fairy tale we all enjoyed several years later. I will also tell you about a miracle that blessed our family in 2012.

Turning back in time even further, I can tell you that it was a phone call in June from Jodi that announced the biopsy results. What was a little lump in Jodi's breast with less than a one percent chance of being malignant was just that. The way we entered Cancerville reminded me of a game I had played as a kid in the Bronx called "tag, you're it." Cancerville had tagged someone we loved; but this was no game. Instead, it was a mind-and-body damaging, life-and-death serious reality.

In response, I sat in the Sloan-Kettering waiting room hoping a terrorist bomb would blow us all up. Why not? Terrorism was happening in the operating room, and we just sat there passively allowing it to occur. At that moment, life had very little meaning as I struggled to picture a happily ever after conclusion.

I wanted to run into the operating room and rip the sharpened scalpel right out of the doctor's hands; but he was just doing his job, and what a job he had. He was trying his very best to save our daughter's life. At that very moment, though, it felt much more like a dirty trick than a treatment. It was a macabre Halloween scene, without costumes or candy. There are so many different, difficult, and dark images that immediately come to our minds when someone we love enters Cancerville. Slowly but surely, you and I will work together to eliminate or minimize them, one by one.

Mark my words, for they are true. When someone you deeply love with all of your heart feels Cancerville's bite, you feel it very strongly too. It is because of your excruciating and, at times, overwhelming emotional pain that I wrote this book. I am confident that my words can help ease your pain and give you a stronger and clearer perspective on how you can contribute to your and your loved one's journey through this harsh place.

There is no denying that Cancerville will test both you and your loved one in ways you could never have imagined. If there is any good news, however, it is that you and your loved one will likely rise to each and every challenge, finding strength neither of you ever knew you had. You can and you will get through this, and I will help you.

In this regard, I admit that I didn't start out the best way. I drank at least five airplane bottles of vodka in the men's room at Sloan-Kettering where I discovered my own BYOB bar. I was hoping to raise my spirits by drinking them. I was at least hoping to slow down my racing mind. The problem was that five bottles weren't enough. Nothing, except perhaps a knockout drug, could diminish the level of anguish I was feeling.

The adrenaline that ran through my body that day more than neutralized the alcohol. The only good thing about finding a bar in a restroom is that you are not very far from a urinal. That benefit notwithstanding, I don't encourage your following my lead. Yet I have a feeling that I am not the first or the last to stumble upon that bar. In fact, "stumble" may be the key word in that sentence.

Let us clearly understand from the beginning that cancer is a formidable foe. In my youth, it was called "the big C" and not discussed. It was almost always a death sentence. Amazing-grace progress has been made over the past fifty years of research, particularly of late.

Cancer is also a complicated set of different diseases. Each type has its own unique issues, prototypes, and protocols, and there are so many unknowns. As people, we crave certainty. We feel better knowing everything will be okay and that our story will have a happily ever after ending. Unfortunately, you don't often get that reassurance in Cancerville. Sometimes, there is no point asking the question because no one has the answer. The easiest case can go wrong and the worst can be fine. I will teach you to give that affirmative reassurance to yourself.

Another scary Cancerville story pushed me to write this book. In June 2010, I received an email from Phil, my friend of almost fifty years. One of his twin eight-year-old grandsons had been diagnosed with a very serious form of leukemia. Cancerville had struck again.

As a psychologist, I am used to hearing bad news in my practice. Caring therapists and counselors tend to cry on the inside as they listen to the sad tales of those they are trying to help. The night I received my friend's scary message, my tears flowed furiously down my cheeks like a saltwater faucet. I was crying because I knew all too well the place he and his family were about to enter. I anticipated their heartache and heartbreak. Once again, those strong feelings that Cancerville can create came rushing back to me. I knew that my friend's family was heading into the bowels of hell and I felt powerless to help them.

From that frustrated sense of impotence, a simple idea came trickling to the surface. On impulse, I sent Rob, my friend's son and father of the stricken boy, an email. I wondered to myself whether I could help guide him through Cancerville as one father who had been there to another who had just entered.

Though I knew Rob and saw him on occasion at family parties, followed his successful career as an attorney with interest, and enjoyed the two novels he had written in his "spare" time, we had no meaningful relationship. He was my friend's son. He, like me, seemed to thrive on being productive, accomplishing goals, and solving problems. Therefore, I suspected he would feel as furiously frustrated as I did in the uncharted and murky waters of Cancerville. I had no idea how, or even if, he would respond to the email that I sent him.

As it turned out, Rob's response was more than encouraging. He said that he had received hundreds of emails since his son had been diagnosed and that he had deleted all of them except the one I sent. He had printed mine out and read it several times a day. That led to an ongoing series of email communications between Rob and me, which helped him travel the obstacle course of Cancerville.

Helping Rob has helped me in many ways. Not only did my emails to him form an outline of what follows, but his positive response to my words of encouragement gave me the confidence and courage to write this book. I have come to realize that I left a piece of me in Cancerville. My communication with

Rob and others in Cancerville, as well as my work on this book, has helped me to reclaim it, like an expensive suit left at the dry cleaners for too long. The good news is that the suit still fits. I wish I could say that about my real suits after six years, but hey, I am working on it. I am pleased to have found this piece of me that I left behind. By writing this book I am not exiting Cancerville, but rather re-entering it with a brand-new view.

That my words helped Rob means that my words may be able to help you as well. Ultimately, that is all we can do in Cancerville—help each other as best we can to get through this most difficult and demanding ordeal. We are all sisters and brothers united by a common bond. Given that the common bond really socks it to us, let's do our personal best to make the best of Cancerville. The words that follow will help you take on Cancerville's challenge, make Cancerville your own, and ultimately own it for the good of your loved one and yourself.

Know that not all professionals agree about promoting positivism in Cancerville. They are concerned about people being unrealistic. They may also be concerned that people will feel that they are "failing" when they can't sustain a hopeful and positive attitude. As you will learn, my beliefs are all based upon a philosophy I call Realistic Optimism. Be aware from the onset that few people can be consistently positive and optimistic in Cancerville or in other complicated situations. People's moods in Cancerville are often in flux and tend to go up and down as events unfold. My goal is to teach you tools that will help you return to neutral or positive feelings whenever you can.

Admittedly, I started out in Cancerville on my hands and knees, kicking and screaming, until I finally figured out that I needed to get to a much more stable place. My years of helping others ultimately helped me to help myself. My simple goal right now is to reach out to you, so I can help you find that positive place more quickly and more often. A hopeful and positive mindset is key to making this very unpleasant experience a little easier to bear.

Now, please reach out and grasp my hand. Though it seems silly, I mean it seriously; indulge me for a very brief moment.

Instead of feeling foolish, try to feel empowered. Every little bit of support helps in Cancerville. Imagine my tight grip leading the way so we can get going. We have a long and demanding journey ahead.

I am firmly convinced that hope is essential in or out of Cancerville; without hope we are lost and doomed to despair, depression, and defeat. As Barbra Streisand so beautifully sang, "Walk on, walk on, with hope in your heart, and you'll never walk alone." As Maya Angelou so beautifully wrote, "Hope slips through the tangle of our fears and evicts despair."

With hope, you and your loved one have a fighting chance—in today's world, a very good chance at that!

William Penzer, Ph.D.
July 8, 2010

An Opening Letter of Hope for Family and Friends ("Heart and Soul Givers") with a Loved One in Cancerville

Dear Family and Friends,

Arriving in Cancerville is a little like getting drafted by the military years ago when you could receive a letter in your mailbox indicating where and when to report to duty. Similarly, without much warning, you are now a green soldier in the boot camp of Cancerville. That is why you need to increase your troop size and strength to help your loved one fight this battle. This book is a manual on how to get through this war zone in one piece. Let me tell you a little more about this war and my book before you proceed.

In many respects, Cancerville is a theater of war. It is, like the battlefields of World War II, the stage upon which a war on cancer is waged. It is where all the action takes place. I wrote these war-related words only to later discover in the comprehensive historical book about cancer, *The Emperor of All Maladies,*[1] by Siddhartha Mukherjee, M.D., Ph.D., that they are not original. Post-WW II pioneers promoting cancer research and seeking funding used the metaphor of a war zone to make their case. Other writers in Cancerville have used this image as well. I neither borrowed the idea nor, as I came to learn, invented it. Sadly, that only underscores the tough nature of this disease. It has been a war zone forever. At least now our medical soldiers are winning more battles.

One theater of this war is behind the scenes, where active research is taking place all over the world. A 2010 *Time* magazine article estimated that in America, $5.6 billion is invested in cancer research every year—more than all other common diseases combined.

In this war zone, highly trained and knowledgeable medical teams join you at cancer centers, hospitals, and private practices around the world. They are the frontline troops in the theater of operations, literally and figuratively. The only difference is that in this war, you and the other troops are not at risk, while your innocent loved one is in the line of fire.

Doctors deploy harsh but powerful ammunition to fight the Cancerville insurgency that has attacked your loved one. As insurgents do, they fight back hard and dirty under the cover of night. This is what can keep you staring at the ceiling at 3 a.m. Please allow me to help you get to sleep at a more reasonable hour. Try to assume that your loved one, with the help of his or her medical team, along with your support, will win this battle.

As for my book/guide/war zone manual, it is often easier to say what something is not about than to describe what something is about. I want to do both so you will know my goals and can decide whether it will be helpful and appropriate for you to continue reading.

This is not a book for those who need to grieve their loss or likely loss in Cancerville. There are many books and other resources to help you do that. Rather, this book was written for those who have reason to believe that there is hope for their loved one. It will support and strengthen your optimism. It will help you find hope at moments when you are feeling none. My words will walk and talk you through this strange and scary place. Together, side-by-side, we will walk the Cancerville beat like a pair of tough street cops in a crime-ridden neighborhood.

This is not a book for those who need to focus on the many details and decisions that you face in Cancerville. If your loved one is young and you need detailed feedback, check out *Living with Childhood Cancer,*[2] by Woznick and Goodheart. That textbook-like opus covers just about everything you can think of relating to Cancerville and then some. It is a compendium of information, complete with many checklists and other useful resources.

If you need that level of detail and your loved one is older, there are many helpful books of that type. It's also important for you to know that this book is not medically based, nor is it filled with data or statistical probabilities. Many books are available that cover that level of medical and scientific detail.

My book is much more the words of a wounded but surviving parent-warrior on the Cancerville battlefield. I have been there, done that, and thrown away the ill-fitting tee shirt. I will help you over the giant emotional speed bumps that will come at you because if ever there was a time for support, this is it. The devil himself could not have designed and built a more diabolical obstacle course.

That said, there is some good news. We humans are amazingly resilient despite all of our doubts, insecurities, and fears. I am hopeful and confident that you will be able to rise to the challenge. Even without this book, you can do that, but in Cancerville you need all the help you can get and I am here to support you. Rest assured that you will be impressed with your own strength and capacity to adapt. You will be equally impressed with those same characteristics demonstrated by your loved one.

My words come right from my heart and head to yours. As we walk the rough and tumble streets of Cancerville together, we may experience a special form of chemistry. We may never meet face-to-face, but I am hopeful that we will develop an empowering relationship that will do Cancerville, yourself, and your loved one proud. I can almost guarantee you that.

This book is not situation specific. No book can take into account the wide range of differences in its population of readers. This is especially true given that cancer cells do not discriminate. They are equal opportunity exploiters. Race, religion, and nationality do not matter to cancer cells; whether one is rich, poor, or somewhere in the middle is also irrelevant. Your loved one may be young, middle-aged, or older. Politically speaking, Cancerville is truly a multi-partisan place. We are all potential targets!

This book speaks to the commonalities that bind us together in our journey through Cancerville. We all have direct lines wirelessly connected from our heads to our hearts, and that is the territory with which I am very familiar and the one I address in this book.

As a psychologist, I strive to simplify rather than to confuse. I will offer you some easy to understand philosophies and ideas that can help you more clearly understand the human mind. These will help you keep yours strong and healthy, despite the pressures of Cancerville. The ammunition you need to fight in the war zone of Cancerville must be lightweight, portable, easy to use, and relieving of your burdens. It needs to be powerful without being heavy.

This is not a book you need to read from cover to cover, so feel free to pick and choose as you like and need. I know that your time and attention are limited in Cancerville. However, the Gestalt school of psychological thought teaches us that "the whole is greater than the sum of its parts." Therefore, if you do have the time, I encourage a full read for more complete and helpful support. In addition, some parts may be more relevant for you, so you may want to revisit them from time to time.

Keep in mind that the reason you don't have to read everything is that there is no test at the end of Cancerville. The test has already begun and I want you to do as well as you can. To do well, you will need to manage, stretch, cope, adapt, be hopeful and positive, and take care of yourself as you support your loved one. This book will help you do all of that and more.

Unlike many self-help books and just about all Cancerville support books, I did not include quotes from famous people at the beginning of each chapter. It would be easy to find relevant ones from Hippocrates to Bernie Siegel, M.D., and many in between that timeline. But I didn't want to imply, by association, that the words of famous people validate mine. Believe me when I say that Hippocrates has not read this book and never will. Neither has Bernie, but hopefully he will, along with many others in the field.

I did opt to begin every chapter with an affirmation to help you validate yourself, which is far more important. View this book as one long letter with me talking to you directly, one Cancerville support to another. In fact, that is precisely what it is. Each chapter builds upon the previous ones and adds another dimension of support. By the conclusion, you will have a comprehensive roadmap guiding you through Cancerville.

In the pages that follow, you will meet many different people who have all been to Cancerville. I have read about some of them and had the pleasure of meeting many others. A few, like Rob and Susan, will pop in and out as we go along. Please know that they are all real people whose experiences, stories, and comments are true without embellishment or editing on my part. In many ways their stories have helped me to better help you.

So, my reader friend, as we embark on our long and winding journey, you will find that we will laugh and cry together. We will walk, at times jog, and occasionally run together. Cancerville is filled with many tall mountains. Together we will climb them with an agility you never knew you had. We might fall off at times, but we will quickly dust ourselves off and slowly, but surely, continue our climb together.

Think of me as an excellent tour guide, umbrella and chin held high, leading you as best as I know how through a place that is not at all excellent. I am hopeful that by following my umbrella, we will be able to make your journey through Cancerville a little easier.

Think of yourself as not only a caregiver, but as a "heart and soul giver" because that is precisely who you are.

Right now, please close your eyes, take a deep breath, and feel my gentle grip leading the way. Trust me that I know the territory well, as I've been here before, sad to say.

Your new Cancerville friend,

Bill

PART I

Getting the Lay of the Land

CHAPTER 1

I will learn how to cope better in Cancerville.

Welcome to Cancerville

It may seem strange to be welcomed to a place where you do not want to be; not wanting to be here is more than understandable. No one volunteers for this assignment, but unfortunately, you are now here. You are going to need to make the most of it in order to be helpful to your loved one and yourself. I wrote this book to help you do just that.

If we are going to engage in a clear and meaningful communication, I will always need to be honest with you. I will never sugarcoat Cancerville, nor its impact and intensity. I will, however, try to be sensitive and supportive in an empowering way. I will help you find ways to smooth Cancerville's rough edges and level the playing field just a bit.

No One Wants to Be in Cancerville

When I first arrived in Cancerville, it was very hard to accept that I was actually there. It took me quite a while to face Cancerville head-on. The reason that people look and are tense, terrified, and teary-eyed in Cancerville is that its streets are dark and mean. Hooligans hang out on every corner and try to make trouble whenever and wherever they can. They have no conscience and show no mercy.

Let's assume the medical team will prevail and beat them one of these days. In the meantime, you need to get ready to rumble and start pumping emotional iron. It is a rough and tumble place. You and your loved one need to be strong to take it on. I assume you will be and do just that.

If you have recently entered this territory, you are probably overwhelmed, exhausted, frightened, and wrestling with a Heinz variety of strong negative emotions. This is to be expected given the lay of the land. Cancerville is a scary place even on a good day. Your challenge is to turn the tables on Cancerville and own it. It will take a little while for you to get there, but rest assured you can and will do just that.

You may have had the disappointing experience of booking a hotel that turned out to be a dump. If so, you most likely tried to move to a better place as soon as possible. As self-protective people, we do our best not to remain in a dump for very long, but sometimes there is no other option available and we have to make the best of a not so pleasant place. That is precisely the case when we are in Cancerville.

No matter how upscale the surroundings in which your loved one receives treatment, it is still in Cancerville. The menu can be three-star, the duvet can be soft and comfortable, and the TV can be a forty-inch HD, but those don't make up for the fact that your loved one is in Cancerville. The likelihood is that the treatment center your loved one is in does not remotely resemble the Ritz; it is probably more like the pits. But that is not important.

What is very important is that the medical team in Cancerville is as dedicated as they come. They will work tirelessly to fight back against the delinquent cells that are the driving force of Cancerville. They want to save your loved one's life just as much as you do, and happily, now more than ever before, they succeed.

The Unpredictability of Cancerville

For most of us, daily life tends to be orderly in many basic ways. Public transportation runs on a published schedule. The garbage in my neighborhood is picked up every Tuesday and Friday, except on major holidays. Traffic lights run predictably except for the occasional outage during an electrical storm or hurricane. This is how the world and we operate. Most people, but for a dare-devilish few, thrive on predictability. Many, if not most of us, require structure, clarity, and reliability to feel "safe" and "in control."

What would it be like if trains, planes, and buses followed no clear schedule or routes? What would life be like if we didn't know what time to arrive for school or work or what time we were supposed to leave? How about not knowing what to expect each day and what was expected of you? I think by now you get my drift. In all of these instances, random and unpredictable forces would create chaos, confusion, and controversy.

Welcome to Cancerville—a very unpredictable place! In Cancerville nothing is certain and just about everything is subject to change without notice. Chemo at 2 a.m.? Maybe. More chemo than anticipated? Probably. A revised treatment plan based upon updated test results, infection, or who knows what? Absolutely possible.

Unfortunately, once your loved one is in Cancerville, you are on a bumpy train that has already left the station. The route and destination are less than clear. All you can do is assume it will finally get to where you want to go so you and your loved one can get off. All of this uncertainty will demand your patience, flexibility, and tolerance for ambiguity. Although these traits may not come naturally, you can acquire them with practice and support. For the moment, grab the strap above your head and hold on tight. Cancerville is a day-at-a-time place, so try to stay focused on the moment without looking too far ahead.

Our Healthy Denial

Cancerville catches us on our blind side like an approaching car not seen in our side or rearview mirrors. We never think that one of our loved ones will be diagnosed with cancer. We have heard others' sad stories, but we exclude that possibility for those we care about and for ourselves.

It's not so different from a horrible head-on crash. We know that life-threatening highway accidents happen all the time, but we never think they will happen to our loved ones or ourselves. This is actually a good thing. If we didn't have this helpful denial mechanism, we would spend much too much time and energy thinking about all of the potential tragedies. We would probably never leave the house, ride in a car, or allow our loved ones to do the same.

It is easier, safer, and healthier for us to use that anticipatory anxiety to take care of our day-to-day responsibilities. So we tend to focus on bills, work issues, kids' school projects, Little League practice, and silly squabbles among family and friends that occasionally crop up. Most people restrict their worries to relatively benign areas of life.

When tragedy, or its potential, leaps out at us like a nightmare, it is a whole different story. We are caught off-guard, become shocked and enraged, and engage in endless "not fair" inner discussions. Whoever said life was fair was probably drunk at the time. I never said it, I swear!

It will take you a while to get past the shock. There is a part of me that still finds it very hard to believe that cancer struck my family, and it has been quite a while now. It is okay to remain shocked, just not shell-shocked. There is no time for that, as you need to be helpful in every possible way.

My hope is that my words will insulate you from the inferno of Cancerville like a racecar driver's fireproof suit. But equally important, I want you to focus on all that you can do to make a difference for your loved one and yourself and on how you can cope with your experience in a much more comfortable way. You need to be more comfortable if you are going to be more comforting.

Everything is Truly Relative

The following is a chart I give to people I help with anxiety, depression, or the like. I call it Penzer's Theory of Relativity. This is not to be confused with the more incomprehensible one by some guy named Einstein, who also started a bagel company.

SEEING THINGS MORE CLEARLY

We need to assess what happens to us along a realistic impact scale:

	1 2	**3 4 5**	**6 7**	**8 9 10**
	Irritation	***Frustration***	***Aggravation***	***Trauma/Tragedy***
Health:	Cold	Flu	Pneumonia	Lung Cancer
Finance:	$50 late fee	$100 late fee	$1000 + loss	Bankruptcy
Accident:	Fender Bender	Car Totaled No Injuries	Head-on Collision With Injuries	Head-on Collision With Death
Work:	Disagreement With Peer	Disagreement With Boss	Poor Evaluation	Fired

The interesting thing about human nature is that we tend to see experiences in the 1 to 4 range as if they were 8 to 10+. This is not only true of the people who visit my colleagues and me, but of most people. There are a few cock-eyed optimists out there, but they are not in the majority. In addition, they all seem to be married to pessimists.

Being in Cancerville slowly changes how we look at and measure life events. We develop a newfound appreciation for these distortions and begin to adjust accordingly. What once seemed oh so important and worrisome now seems oh so silly. You will keep running into these interpretive shifts, and at some point you will begin to wish for the lower level stresses you once dreaded. Nonetheless, here you are, much as you didn't expect to and don't want to be.

I am a great believer in the strength, courage, and perseverance that people bring to the battlefields of their lives. I have had the privilege of repeatedly observing that in my office all these years. I am also a great believer in the power of words that feed and fuel those very characteristics. My sincere belief is that what follows are powerful words to help you cope a little better in the place I have come to call Cancerville.

Take a very deep breath, let it out very, very slowly, and then do it again. Our journey is about to begin. You may have already started, but I've only just joined your team. Welcome to Cancerville—one hell of a place!

In Sum

Cancerville has many rough and bumpy roads on which we have to travel. It reminds me of the difficult and unpredictable terrain I encountered in East Africa where many boulders and rocks blocked the unpaved roads. Though you may have to go into the emotional equivalent of four-wheel drive, you will make it through. The good news is that your loved one and you can, and likely will, rise to the challenge of being in Cancerville with strength, courage, and dignity. As you keep reading, my goal is to help make your journey easier and smoother.

It took me a while to figure out that I was not as powerless as I felt. Let's move on so I can help you realize that you have much more power than you think you do right now.

CHAPTER 2

I will be a helpful support to my loved one.

Converting Rapidly from Powerless to Powerful

I don't care how important you are, how much clout you have, or how much money you have accumulated. I don't care if your name is Gates, Trump, Kennedy, or Winfrey. You might have the financial resources to buy an organ for your loved one, a private room, or a Medevac plane to fly to a different cancer center. Once there, however, you will feel as powerless as the rest of us.

The Power of Love

One of the most common feelings among family in Cancerville, most especially parents, is that they are not doing their job properly. They feel they are not able to protect their child or loved one. Parents are used to kissing the boo-boo and magically making it all better. Unfortunately, those magic kisses alone don't improve your loved one's medical condition in Cancerville. Most of the medical magic rests solely with your medical team. Yet, magical or otherwise, hugs and kisses can make miracles happen in Cancerville when it comes to emotional support and healing. At times, positive attitudes and warm and loving support have been found to contribute to strengthening immune systems and helping to overcome a variety of medical problems in and out of Cancerville.

Bernie Siegel, M.D. wrote a landmark book in the late 1980's called *Love, Medicine and Miracles.*[3] In that book, Siegel repeatedly stresses the importance of emotional support in the healing and recovery process. He is a strong believer in the power of the patient and his or her family to facilitate healing. He is a lobbyist for love as being a potent force in the recovery process. He states, "I am convinced that unconditional love is the most powerful known stimulant of the immune system... The truth is love: heals."

That a surgeon was able to realize and communicate the important influence of loving support in serious health arenas points to him being a very special person and a unique physician. He was also part of the movement that championed the doctor and "exceptional" patient as partners in the medical process. Although the medical field is not so "I/Thou" today as it once was, there is still room for improvement in this area. This will be addressed in Chapter 6, "Meetings With the Dedicated Doctors."

The medical side of Cancerville is exactly where you may feel a sense of powerlessness. You are capable of influencing your loved one's attitude, spirit, and hopefulness, but not the disease itself. Without the ability to provide medical or magical interventions, you may feel that you are unable to make a difference, as if weakened by a special form of kryptonite. As we will see, this belief is technically true, but irrelevant. The love and support you can bring to your loved one is just as important and valuable as what the doctors can do on the medical side. Blended together, emotional support and medical treatment form a very powerful healing partnership. Please reread that last sentence!

The Illusion of Family Protectiveness

Realistically, a parent's ability to protect his or her child in a host of life circumstances is more illusion than reality. Parents need to believe in their protective powers to avoid and deny the real and present dangers that exist. The same, by the way, is true for other family members and even friends.

Parents and other relatives can certainly take care of infants not equipped to take care of themselves. They can oversee colds, sore throats, bronchitis, broken limbs, croup, and other relatively minor illnesses. Of course, parents hold their children's little hands until these young people are able to navigate streets and parking lots by themselves.

Caring family members also try to soothe a child's hurt feelings when the neighbor kid or a classmate does something insensitive. They do the same when a child strikes out in a Little League game or fails a test at school. We are able to apply the physical and emotional equivalent of first aid to our loved ones, but there are many life events beyond our influence or control.

The following list may seem extreme, but it will help you understand why I feel that parents, family, and friends are not always well-positioned to help or protect their loved ones:

- Columbine-type incidents
- terrorist attacks
- physical and/or emotional abuse
- car, bus, train, plane, and boat crashes
- fires
- Mother Nature's violent side
- drownings
- gangs and bullies
- animal attacks

- drug overdoses
- other life-threatening diseases

Need I say more? Every day, in every place in the world, serious stuff happens that can hurt, maim, or kill a loved one. Cancerville is just another place where our direct protective powers are limited.

As if to prove this point, forty-three-year-old Kevin, a good man I have known for many years, recently drowned in a freak scuba diving accident along with a female friend. In the past seven months, nine people have died in scuba related accidents in the Florida Keys. That number is surprising given the many safeguards that are built into that sport.

Taking Action in Cancerville

Unless you are an oncologist, you can't cure your loved one. As you will discover, however, there are many things you can and will do to help ease and brighten your loved one's day and stay in Cancerville. You can and will provide a wide variety of support services. These are as important as the medical ones. When medical and emotional supports are combined, they form a strong tag team to wrestle cancer to the ground. If you don't believe me, just ask Bernie!

Notwithstanding our limited powers of protection, we can all do some amazing things for our loved ones. As we shall see, they need not be major. In many ways little things mean a lot in Cancerville. I am convinced, however, that taking action is exactly what takes us from feeling powerless to powerful. The faster you can do that, the better you will feel.

I want to share two stories that reflect exceptional action that was taken in Cancerville. I would not expect you, most people, or even myself to duplicate such Herculean efforts. These stories, however, are inspiring and will hopefully propel you forward in your own unique way. Then I will share with you my own experience taking action in Cancerville that shows how a simple gesture unexpectedly helped my daughter.

Taking Action to Influence the World

An excellent example of someone making a powerful contribution not only to her family but also to the world is Nancy Brinker. If you are not familiar with her name, I understand, as I was not either until very recently. Her identity will come more clearly into focus if I tell you that her sister's name was Susan G. Komen. Nancy promised Susan she would make a difference in raising people's awareness of breast cancer. And my goodness, has she ever lived up to that promise!

Sadly, Susan died from breast cancer at the age of thirty-six. Nancy, herself a breast cancer survivor at the age of thirty-seven, went on to found an organization that fulfilled her promise to her sister. Not only has her "Susan G. Komen for the Cure" organization raised over one-and-a-half billion dollars, but also, and as importantly, it has raised awareness of this disease around the world.

For these and many other accomplishments, Nancy was presented with the Presidential Medal of Freedom in 2009 and recently wrote a book called *Promise Me: How a Sister's Love Launched the Global Movement to End Breast Cancer.*[4] In every way possible and then some, Nancy Brinker has modeled taking action in Cancerville.

Please do not try to measure your contributions against hers. She is a very unique woman who was driven to make a difference by upholding her promise to her sister. She has organizational, communication, and marketing skills that are not widely distributed in our population. She was also married to a very capable and successful businessman who, among other things, founded the Chili's restaurant chain. There are many other stories around the world of people turning their grievous personal losses into caring "winnings" for others.

My references to outstanding and exceptional actions in response to Cancerville are meant to help move you forward, rather than trying to encourage you to compete with such Cancerville champions. Remember, even simple, loving actions can mean a lot.

One Man's Action-Packed Effort for His Family

Sometimes we have to accept delegating our "control" to others while we work on the sidelines to do all we can to be there for our loved one. No one taught me this lesson better than Rob, whose young son Jake was diagnosed with leukemia. Thankfully, Jake is now in remission.

Rob is a man who has always made things happen in his life. What he made happen for his ill son and his healthy twin son, Chase, is quite impressive. Here is a partial list:

- created a team that numbered in the hundreds, if not more, that helped on every level in every way, including prayer vigils around the world
- worked with the school to get support, help, and tutorials for both of his sons
- obtained signed jerseys for his sons from hometown national sports teams and even a hospital visit from some local heroes
- had a constant village of visitors when his son was hospitalized at Sloan-Kettering for an extended period of time
- had local restaurants name burgers and fries after his sons as a way to collect money for cancer research
- organized a walk with the help of family that raised over $60,000 for childhood leukemia research
- communicated with pediatric oncologists at two other major cancer centers, St. Jude Children's Research Hospital and Children's Hospital of Pennsylvania, to make sure they agreed with the treatment protocol at Sloan-Kettering.
- rallied the support of both sides of his and his wife's family to an incredible extent
- contacted children's TV programs and got autographed pictures
- had many, many people donate toys, not only for his son, but for other children at the hospital, as well

- drove the "bus" daily back and forth from Westchester, New York to Manhattan, which takes a good hour-plus each way
- set up a video chat between Jake and his school friends when the school would not do it for "legal" reasons
- wrote daily blogs to vent his feelings and frustrations and to bring family and friends up to date on what was happening

I'm probably leaving out so many other areas that Rob tapped into to help his sons directly and indirectly, to raise people's awareness of the devastation of Cancerville, and to raise money for the good of the cause. Rob literally left no stone unturned. Clearly, he had many available resources and a powerful team surrounding him and his family.

Few, myself included, possess the ability to do so much. Each of you, however, will do some important things for the good of your loved one. I offer Rob's accomplishments as an example of what a few people are able to do in Cancerville. Please do not measure yourself against his impressive list. Measure yourself against your list of helpful accomplishments. Cancerville is not a competitive event or a reality TV show. It is a realistic challenge to which, I am confident, you will rise in your own way.

Interestingly enough, Rob is quick to admit that, despite all of his major efforts, what pleased Jake most was a simple gift. Rob gave him a necklace that Jake had always admired. It belonged to Jake's great-grandfather, and they had been very close until his great-grandfather passed. Wearing this necklace comforted him and gave him strength and support during this very difficult time. Like the song goes, "Little Things Mean A Lot."

Taking Action to Help Our Daughter

When Jodi was being treated, my wife and I flew back and forth from Ft. Lauderdale, Florida to New York City many, many times. We wanted to meet with the doctors, be there for Jodi's surgery and chemo treatments, and bring support and occasional fun to the scene. I think we saw almost every show on Broadway. We were there to celebrate special days. Though we could not be there every day, we were fortunate to be able to be there every time we wanted or needed to be. There were daily phone calls as well. In today's wired world, some of these calls could have been made via Skype, so we could have been "face-to-face."

The only thing we couldn't do was take over Jodi's cancer cells by proxy, although we would have if that had been possible. I know you would, too, as a parent, grandparent, or loving partner, but it just doesn't work that way.

Though Ronnie or I could not eliminate the cancer or soothe our daughter's physical wounds, we tried our best to help heal the emotional ones. We also helped organize prayers for her all around the world. It is interesting how Cancerville can convert "non-believers," if not into "true-believers," then at least into "it's worth-a-try-believers." You just never know what prayer can do!

It took me a while to realize just how powerful we all were despite our initial sense of powerlessness. The best way to deal with and overcome a sense of helplessness and powerlessness is, as I have said, to take action. The more that you can do, the better you will most likely feel. There was nothing that you could have done to prevent your loved one from entering Cancerville. However, there is much that you can do to be helpful once your loved one is there.

Your support doesn't always have to be something major or even expensive. It can be a simple act of kindness and love. The day of Jodi's surgery, after she was back in her room, I needed to get out and escape briefly from Cancerville's New York headquarters. I needed some fresh air to clear my mind, and I probably needed another drink, but that's beside the point. I am not particularly proud of sometimes using alcohol to offset my pain, but in some situations, you've just got to do what you've got to do. On occasion, we humans, smart as we might be, can be pretty dumb. Guilty as charged!

So I went for a walk and wandered into the megastore Bed Bath and Beyond. There was no booze there despite all the B's.

I needed to get Beyond, but all I got was Bed and Bath. A few minutes into the store, I saw a small pink pillow with arm and leg-like appendages that vaguely resembled a person. I instinctively bought it and brought it back to give to Jodi. I later learned that she slept with the pillow at night and sometimes took it in the car with her to cushion the literal bumps in the road on the Manhattan streets. I was completely unaware that it helped her with the figurative bumps as well.

Years later, I received an email from Jodi telling me that she had to retire "Pinky" because he had pretty much come undone: "Better him than my daughter!" I thought. She shared how attached she had become to him and how much he had helped her get through those troubled times.

I was struck and touched that a simple $9.99 purchase could have had such a significant impact on her. Being a psychologist, I wondered to myself whether it wasn't so much "Pinky" as it was that I gave it to her on what was the very worst day of her life. Maybe what "Pinky" represented beyond his cushiness was my comforting and cushioning support and loving presence beside my daughter at those times when I wasn't able to be there in person. I'd really like to believe that.

We just never know the impact that our words, actions, or small gifts will have on our loved ones. It is important for you to remember that sometimes it doesn't take much to make a significant difference. Just a loving hug and kind word, or the equivalent of a "Pinky" at the right moment, can be significant.

In Sum

After reading this chapter, I hope you come away realizing that you are not as weak or powerless in Cancerville as you might think or feel. You see, the kryptonite really only applies to the medical side. You are not expected to be a superman or superwoman in that zone. Leave that to the super doctors.

There is so much you are doing right now and that you will continue to do to make a difference for your loved one and, in turn, for yourself. Of that I am very confident. My confidence comes from the fact that, among other things, you are reading this book. Bravo!

In Chapter 9, you will learn what a pride bank deposit is, so that each step of the way you can fill yours to the top. Doing helpful things and taking action for your loved one definitely adds to your pride bank and helps you feel and cope better generally, and especially in Cancerville.

Let's move on to talk about adapting to this most demanding place. It is a challenge, but one I am hopeful you will take on with confidence, strength, and some moxie as well.

CHAPTER 3

I am an adaptive person and have a track record to prove that.

Striving to Adapt to a Place from which You Really Want to Run

If taking action helps you to overcome your sense of powerlessness in Cancerville, then a variety of specific actions and attitudinal adjustments will help you to better adapt to its demands. To demonstrate your power, you will need to adapt to Cancerville by finding ways to be a supportive, loving, and contributing member of the team. All animals are programmed to adapt to their environs, as well as to significant shifts in the terrain. In my humble opinion, none is better suited to that process and goal-directed purpose than human beings. You will adapt to Cancerville; I have no doubt about that!

People Rise to the Challenge

Catastrophes and crises create chaos, which in turn demands immediate adjustments. Entering Cancerville is obviously a crisis of grand proportion, but one that you will ultimately manage. As people, we adapt naturally and automatically to life's demands. Think of times in the past when you had to cope with and adjust to difficult situations. Reminding yourself how you were able to do it then will help you gain confidence that you can do it again now.

In speaking about crises, I vividly remember November 22, 1963. It was one month to the day before Ronnie and I were to be married, and I was nervous enough! I was teaching a class at New York University as a graduate assistant. A pained voice came over the loudspeaker announcing that President John F. Kennedy had been shot in Dallas, Texas. Everyone stood up and left the room; I didn't even have to say, "Class dismissed." I opened my mouth but no words came out. Like everyone else that day, I made my way home in a daze.

As word spread of Kennedy's assassination, the world as we knew it changed. People spent the next several days watching events unfold, glued to their tiny black and white TVs. The same, of course, occurred on 9/11. Hardly anyone went to work that day or for days after, and once again, time stood still. I can't recall how many times I watched the color footage of the planes crashing into the World Trade Center before I just couldn't bear to watch anymore.

Those painful news images are really no different from the announcement that cancer cells have invaded your loved one's body; it is hard not to replay that news over and over again in your head. However, I will teach you ways to stop doing that in Part IV of this book.

Such Cancerville news related to your loved one is a clarion call to arms; the chaos that ensues, emotionally and otherwise, is unprecedented. The announcement that your loved one has cancer is nothing short of your own private assassination and 9/11 combined! Your world, as you have come to know it, is dramatically and traumatically changed. It will require major shifts in your routines, priorities, thoughts, and attitudes.

Yet, unlike national catastrophes, Cancerville is not for spectators. It won't be on TV and most people will have no idea what you are going through. Many with loved ones in Cancerville report feeling very alone, even if they have a support team around them. Try to remind yourself that you are actually part of a very large network—in America, one and a half million people are diagnosed with cancer every year. You are an integral and essential part of your loved one's team. In some instances, you may be the only member of the team—but you are not alone.

When Cancerville hits, all of a sudden and out of the blue, you are faced with confusions, questions, major decisions, and logistical adjustments that resemble a space shuttle launch. Yet the likelihood is that you don't have the support team or personnel of NASA. You will start creating a support structure and team out of whatever material and "personnel" are on hand. Creatively taking action, moving slowly forward, researching, learning, and supporting will all help you and your loved one to move ahead into calmer terrain.

The Process of Adapting

Adaptation is an interesting and understudied human experience. The majority of people do it naturally and automatically; necessity is truly the mother of invention. I have repeatedly observed people rise to the challenges of life and of Cancerville. There are only a very few who fall by the wayside. Make up your mind now that you will figure it out as you go along. Your loved one needs you to be there, strong and present. You need to be there for yourself as well.

This all makes me think of my mother and myself when my father died of a heart attack in 1960, at age forty-nine. After my father's passing, my mom and I adapted. We tightened our belts and she went from part-time to full-time work. I also found a part-time job while attending college full-time.

My father's death left emotional scars on my mom and me, but we coped as best we could and learned over time to accept the painful reality of his loss. Counseling or support groups back then were not readily available. We just sucked it up and moved forward.

Even a successful outcome in Cancerville will leave emotional scars. But remember, nobody dies from those scars. Sometimes, you can even learn from them. I know that my mother and I just kept marching on. I haven't stopped yet, and she only did after having lived to one hundred. In Chapter 22, we will look at some of the positive life lessons one can learn in Cancerville.

In all zones of our lives, much as most of us do not enjoy change, we adapt to it. We suck it up, stare challenges in the face, and do what we have to do. We certainly don't like Cancerville. No— wait a minute here—we absolutely hate it! Be aware, my wife edited out the word I originally had before "hate." I still feel that I should put it back in. Please do that on your own. We do, however, whatever Cancerville asks and expects of us and try our best to do it with a smile, simply because our loved one needs that warmth. The demands of Cancerville act as a lubricant for change and adaptation. What makes people so special is our ability to do just that.

I believe adaptation is a slow but steady process of determining what is needed and reacting accordingly. It is a fluid and often changing experience that goes with the flow of what is happening in the moment. Therefore, I do not see what follows as steps (as in one, two, etc.), but rather as components to foster your adaptation to Cancerville.

Acceptance

A most important component of adaptation involves your acceptance of the situation. This includes getting past the initial shock and realizing that "it is my loved one's turn," hard as that may be to believe. Clearly, all of our beliefs regarding immunity from harm's way are false and illusory.

I know you would like to run with your loved one out of Cancerville to a much safer and calmer place. Let's assume you will, but not just yet. Acceptance allows you to mobilize your energies and target them directly to address your loved one's needs. It also helps you to realize that you are in the safest place you can be under these circumstances. Much support and many medical treatments are available for your loved one in Cancerville.

Awareness

Generally speaking, people vary with regard to their need for information. That is true, as well, for family and friends who have a loved one in Cancerville. Some want to know everything about their loved one's condition. They read and research till all hours of the night. Others prefer to learn some of the details and leave it at that. Another group of people in Cancerville prefer to learn about their loved one's treatment plan, but not much else.

All three approaches are fine; it just depends on personality and comfort level. Regardless of how much information you seek, you will gain a clearer sense of what your loved one and you will be facing in the weeks and months ahead. Please keep in mind that there is no "right way" to journey through Cancerville. Follow any approach that feels comfortable and appropriate for you. We are fortunate to be living at a time when information gathering is easier than ever. Having said that, we need to be cautious and always consider the source.

Attitude Adjustment

Adjusting and readjusting your attitude is a most important component of your adaptation. My hope is that, as we walk through Cancerville together, you will be able to embrace a stronger, healthier, and more positive mindset as quickly as possible. Though I personally experienced a full range of negative feelings as I entered Cancerville, I came to realize that such feelings were hurtful and toxic to my family and myself. I wasted too much time and energy by feeling sorry for my family's plight. That time and energy could have been better directed toward a more accepting and optimistic approach. As I have said, adaptation is a process with a slow learning curve. I hope to help you avoid the thinking traps into which I fell—headfirst.

Action

In a most interactive way, all of the above components flow into your accomplishing the goals you set to be a helpful, loving, and supportive resource. It is the Nike "Just Do It!" theme personified. It requires the same type of commitment that you have made in other goal-directed areas of your life. Most people tend to do all they can and all they need in many areas, but most especially when it comes to their loved ones. It is unlikely that those who don't do all they can for their loved ones would even be reading this book.

As I have said in other writings in a variety of contexts, love is a verb that demands action, consistency, and commitment. It is far, far more than a greeting card. In Cancerville, your love may be the most powerful and versatile "tool" you have and can be used in many different and helpful ways. Your warm smile, hug, kiss, pat on the back, reassurances, and kind words of support and encouragement are a special type of emotional "medicine."

A Never Ending Commitment

Much research has shown that, in a variety of adverse situations, persistence wins out. Much can be said for plodding patiently but powerfully along with a "can do" attitude and a "will do whatever it takes" set of beliefs. In life, there are those who say "uncle" and those who say "never!" In Cancerville, you need to be part of the latter group.

Strength is often measured in the long run—literally and figuratively. People who persevere usually accomplish their goals and achieve their dreams, simply because they don't give up. The significant things in life are almost never achieved easily. Much needs to be pursued doggedly, at least for a while. Think of athletes, Olympic or otherwise; they have logged thousands upon thousands of hours doing difficult and demanding things to achieve their goals and to fulfill their dreams. They have sweated it out just as you are now doing.

See yourself becoming a Cancerville athlete and going the distance for your loved one. As you do, you will adapt faster and easier to its demands. You will begin to see it as another important challenge in your life, similar, but more daunting, to others you have faced and overcome.

Wrestling with the Logistics of Cancerville

On a practical basis, the shifts and adaptations you will need to make in Cancerville will depend on your relationship to your loved one. You may be reading this as the parent of a young child, teen, or adult child, or you may be a spouse or partner. You may be an adult child or sibling, or you may be a cousin or a former college roommate who lives far away. The following chart roughly sketches the level of adaptation that you will likely need to make, depending upon the specifics:

INCREASING LEVELS OF ADAPTATION, CHANGE, AND RESPONSIBILITY

1	2	3	4	5	6	7	8	9	10
remote relatives / friends			***geographically closer friends***		***geographically closer relatives***			***immediate family / partners***	

Obviously, there are no hard and fast rules in Cancerville. The independent adult child with cancer may have to temporarily come back to his or her parents' home to live. Parents or grandparents may have to temporarily move in to manage their loved one's household. There is no denying that young children in Cancerville require families to make the most logistical adjustments, especially if they are treated inpatient and, most especially, if there are other young siblings.

In addition, even those who are geographically remote may choose to visit and become part of the team. Jodi's close high school and college friends realized that her chemo and compromised immune system would prevent her from flying to Atlanta, Georgia to attend their annual summer reunion. So they all flew to New York for a weekend of fun and frolic. I know how special that was for her, as well as for my wife and me.

There are many instances when friends provide support and help as well. The story I will soon share about Linda shows her concern and caring for a family member and for a friend. My graphic, computer, video, and all around helper, Brad, told me that the grandchild of a family friend had recently been diagnosed with leukemia. Brad and his wife spent a great deal of time searching the web and finding Facebook pages of relevant support organizations. No one asked them to do that, but they wanted to reach out and help in any way they could. It makes a significant and heart-warming difference when other people stretch and sacrifice to be there as sources of support.

As the previous chart shows, immediate family members typically absorb the bulk of the responsibilities by making the greatest shifts to their schedules. All of a sudden, work, play, social events, exercise, and the like are put on hold or reduced to limited participation. These activities are often replaced by the requirements of Cancerville. Doctor appointments and meetings, treatments, recuperation from treatments, information gathering, and cheer-up support for your loved one all take center stage and become the priority for an indefinite period of time.

Much as many of us are creatures of habit, we are also able to quickly shift and do whatever is required of us. Thank goodness for that. Being my own boss made it a lot easier to adjust my schedule so that we could be there for Jodi's treatments.

Most bosses are flexible and understanding of the demands and shifts that Cancerville imposes upon family members.

Without realizing it, we constantly adapt and plan in order to effectively manage our lives. Think of all the planning and work that goes into the simple goal of having a family picnic. Cancerville, a place where we do not have much experience, certainly requires even more strategic planning. Cancerville is no picnic and no fun whatsoever! Nonetheless, a strategic plan needs to be established. This forms the basis for your adapting to its demands.

Logistical, financial, attitudinal, and emotional issues need to be thought over and discussed. For example, what needs to be done to mobilize the medical insurance? Who will take your loved one to chemo appointments? What do you need to do to set up necessary schedule changes? Lines of communication all around need to be created. A great deal of planning needs to go into how to approach and ultimately take charge in Cancerville.

There is also a need for Plan B if Plan A doesn't seem to be working the way your loved one needs. In all serious areas of life, there needs to be a back-up plan. Rob's Plan A was a children's cancer hospital in Westchester, New York, not far from his and his family's homes. Plan B was Sloan-Kettering, a mecca of treatment in Manhattan, New York. It was much less convenient but much more reassuring to be at a center like that, which is why he went with Plan B.

Susan flew from Ft. Lauderdale, Florida to MD Anderson Cancer Center in Houston, Texas for a Monday morning appointment when the chemo protocols that were tried at her local treatment center had not yielded results. She had also been to Moffitt Cancer Center in Tampa, Florida. In Cancerville, one often searches for the "best" physician, place, program, or protocol. You can support your loved one's choice to do that as part of adapting to a complicated situation.

An Example of Someone Truly Being There

Linda modeled just how well a caring person can adapt to some of Cancerville's unique demands and be there for a loved one. She did that when her dad was diagnosed with terminal lung cancer, a likely result of being a heavy smoker all his life. She was there for him in every possible way—logistically, emotionally, and financially. She was a gracefully flowing fountain of support, even stretching beyond her own comfort zone in the process.

Of note is that one of her Dad's only pleasures was playing slot machines. It made him happy to sit in the casino for hours on end, smoke cigarettes, and play the machines, all the while chasing the elusive winning combinations.

Linda took her dad to doctor appointments, went to his home to help her stepmom, and encouraged her dad during difficult times. In addition, she gave him a large daily slot stipend with which to play and arranged for rides to and from the casino. When no one else was available, she drove him herself. "I want him to spend his last months of life doing what he enjoys and what gives him pleasure," she once told me. She didn't judge his habit; she just supported his "hobby." He did pass, but until the very end when he just couldn't get to the casino, he "cachinged" his way to heaven smiling all the way. Linda smiled, as well, and considered it one of her best investments—not financially, but emotionally.

There is, however, another turn of the tale. A few years after her father passed, Linda's best friend was diagnosed with cancer. Linda jumped right in with her whole self—again—and became a solid and helpful resource. She was there for moral support, helped fight for medical insurance, attended just about every doctor appointment and chemo treatment, and helped her in every way possible, bringing Cindy loyalty, love, laughter, and lunch wherever they went. In fact, post-surgery, she invited Cindy to stay at her house for several days of support and TLC.

The helper role is not always relegated to relatives, as there are times when friends play a very important and special part too. Who of us couldn't use a Linda in our lives? The question remains, how many of us can model her wonderfully kind, generous, and loving support? I am optimistic that readers of this book will do just that, each in their own unique and special ways.

In Sum

It is likely that you will have to make many adjustments in order to adapt to the demands of Cancerville. All of a sudden, schedules and routines are turned upside down. What once seemed important and of high priority to you might become insignificant, as Cancerville will likely become the main event and your primary focus. Your survival and that of your loved one matters, but not much else feels all that significant.

You will learn how to leap those tall buildings, if not in a single bound, in two, three, or more, as needed. You will pick up whatever emotional kryptonite invades your mind and fling it into another stratosphere far from Cancerville. You may have to do that over and over, but you will each time it presents itself. Your loved one needs your strong and unwavering support, and I suspect that you are fit for the role. If not, I will help you get there.

You will be able to make the necessary logistical adaptations no matter what they are. The challenge will be for you to rise to the attitudinal and emotional adjustments. Please keep reading, as you will find much support for those challenges as we continue through Cancerville together.

It is very important that right from the beginning you lower the spotlight on catastrophe. Our minds automatically go for "worst-case scenarios." Let's see if, in the next chapter, I can help you learn to go to "better-case scenarios."

CHAPTER 4

My loved one will be a survivor.

Turning Down the Spotlight on Catastrophe

As soon as you hear a diagnosis of cancer, your first thought is that "I am going to lose my loved one." Obviously, there is a very powerful association between being in Cancerville and death. Many cancer patients have told me that nothing awakens one's sense of mortality as much as a cancer diagnosis. Susan said, "It's like getting hit in the face with a mortality pie and it doesn't taste good." The same raised consciousness is true for those close to the patient.

Nonetheless, I want you to try to lose any thoughts of losing your loved one. The only way to exist comfortably in Cancerville is to be "balls to the walls" positive. That goes for females too. I believe that both males and females have them and women's are invisible, but bigger. Repeat these words every day: "Cancer can be cured!"

There is little room for doubt, even if others' words, books, research, or statistics feed into fearful feelings. Instead, try to leave your fears out of the emotional equation. Although this will be good for your own mental health, I encourage you to do so for your loved one's benefit too. Oftentimes, your loved one can read your feelings without you saying a word. One of your many goals is to encourage hopefulness and optimism.

Many who were told they had a limited time to live are still alive and well years later. For example, my friend Tom was told his leukemia would take him out of the game within six to twelve months. He was supposed to be the late Tom back in the late 1980's. All these years later, he still smiles about beating that dire prediction.

Renowned psychologist and researcher, Martin Seligman, Ph.D., said it best. In his book *Learned Optimism* he states,[5] "Life inflicts the same setbacks and tragedies on the optimist as on the pessimist, but the optimist weathers them better... Even when things go well for the pessimist he is haunted by forebodings of catastrophe." Seligman's research reminds us of the value of being positive-minded, and his writings can help us to become more optimistic. You will hear more about his work in Chapter 11, which encourages positive self-talk.

Illusions of Safety and Predictability

In Chapter 2, I spoke about parents' illusions of being able to protect their children. I listed examples of the many dangers that threaten our loved ones every day. How many of you, by a show of hands, will lie awake worrying that your home and loved ones will burn to the ground tonight? I see only one man's hand raised, and I'm happy to say he is in therapy.

Yet this terrible misfortune happens many times every day somewhere or other. House fires, car accidents, assaults, and abductions happen to random families. Mother Nature periodically shows her wrath in many devastating ways. Clearly,

Cancerville does not have a monopoly on taking your loved one from you. There are many paths to heaven, only one of which is cancer.

You can't predict outcomes in life or in Cancerville. After all, if you were really good at predicting the future, you would be a billionaire by now and not too many of us can claim that title. In reality, most people, including myself, have amazing hindsight and limited foresight. So what makes us think that we can predict outcomes in a place as complicated as Cancerville? We are much better off believing that somehow or other our loved one will walk the maze of Cancerville and ultimately escape alive. We do need to be realistic in this regard, which will be discussed in more detail in Chapter 10, "Embracing a Really Simple Philosophy: Realistic Optimism."

Obviously, walking around Cancerville fearing your loved one's premature demise is, quite frankly, an exercise in self-torture. This fear serves no useful purpose other than to inflict pain, torment, and high levels of anxiety. These will not serve you or your loved one well. If you could convince me that your personal torment would alleviate your loved one's suffering, then I would be all for it. But since this isn't the case, please do your best to reduce the candlepower of that spotlight.

I have sold hope with the tenacity of a drug dealer my entire career. Not only has it helped people free themselves from their inner torments, but it has also paid multiple dividends. Being positive, hopeful, and optimistic generates more of those same feelings. Those feelings can, in turn, increase your energy to tackle whatever challenges you face in the future. In the same way, fostering hope in Cancerville will help you make better decisions for yourself and your loved one.

On Loss

People don't like to lose—ever! I can recall playing indoor racquetball for many years until my angioplasty in 2001 prematurely ended my competitive fun. Before I had to hang up my racquetball outfits and give away my racquet, I played as if I was going to win a gold medal, rather than just trying to beat a friend or neighbor.

Even today, I do not like to lose a silly board game, even when playing with my grandchildren. My Bronx Yankees played for the pennant in 2010. Even though my serious fan days are long gone, I didn't want them to lose. They did lose, however, despite their well-paid roster, and I was disappointed. We humans are seemingly programmed to root, root, root for the home team, even in situations without great significance or meaning.

If seemingly irrelevant losses can be upsetting, we rapidly realize how the possible loss of a loved one can be so devastating. I am not denying the seriousness of the situation. I am not insensitive to your innermost fears. I am simply trying to teach you a lesson that took me a while to learn. Your fear of losing your loved one needs to be bypassed via emotional open-heart surgery so that you can endure your experience in Cancerville. There is just no time or energy for such torment. You need to table the notion of anything other than survival for your loved one. This book is intended to help you do just that.

Assuming Survival

In the final analysis, you just never know how the story will conclude until you get there. So don't sell your loved one or the army of protectors in Cancerville short. Assume and embrace the enduring belief that your loved one will live and become a survivor, just like the millions of people who are part of that strong group. Believe that your loved one will spit in the face of the ugly cancer cells, survive the ordeal, and get back to his or her life all the stronger for squarely facing the challenge of Cancerville and for overcoming it.

During Jodi's treatment time in Cancerville, I would often say to myself: "The world could end tomorrow or the next day and we would all be gone, so I won't worry about my daughter anymore than I worry about that." I worked very hard to keep turning down the spotlight on my fear of losing my daughter.

One of the ways I did this was by reminding myself of many other potential dangers, such as those I listed in the previous chapter, which I don't usually worry about regarding my loved ones or myself. I again became reacquainted with how fragile human life is, both in and out of Cancerville. I also came to appreciate and feel a full measure of gratitude for every day.

As if to highlight and underscore my thoughts, my friend Ben called me after Jodi began chemo. He said, "Billy, I envy you." I said, "How can that be Benjy? I told you what's going on and I am miserable about Jodi." He said, "I am much more miserable. My daughter, Jessica, who just turned eighteen, was taken from us last night in a horrific car accident. She was an innocent passenger sitting in the backseat. At least Jodi has a chance, a good chance." I rest my case about life and death, Cancerville, and all the other vile "villes" that can hurt our loved ones.

That you and your loved one are alive at this very moment is what matters. All of the rest is unknown. Yours could be a sorrowful ending or a positive one. Why not assume that like ours, yours will be a happy one too, and root, root, root for your loved one.

I encourage you to think beyond Cancerville to a time in the future when you and your loved one's lives return to what some call a "new normal." Picture a calmer, quieter, less stressful time. See routine returning. Believe that you and your loved one's nightmare will conclude and that he or she will be a cancer survivor.

Most minds, not just yours or mine, tend to gravitate toward negative anticipations. I would like you to try to block yours from going there and to try to make positive and hopeful assumptions. If this is too large a jump for your mind to make, then at least strive for neutral. Say to yourself: "Self, I don't know what the future will bring. I will wait and see and try to assume we will all be okay." That's all you can really do.

At a recent meeting, I met up with Malcolm, whose adult son was going through chemo at the same time as Jodi. We were acquaintances who, unfortunately, were going through Cancerville as fathers of adult children. He and I used to email back and forth late into the night to try to give each other support. I'm pretty sure he was more helpful to me than I was to him.

He still painfully remembers the hospital vigil during which his son was burning up with fever. At that time, his son's lymphoma had returned, requiring a second harsh round of chemo. When we recently met he told me, "Those were scary times for my wife and me, and for my son, his wife and kids. But we always believed he would survive and be okay. And now it is four years after that second rough round of chemo and he is doing fine."

In the middle of Cancerville, if things get really mean and scary as they did for this man and his family, it can be hard to imagine that the outcome could actually be okay. Yet over and over we see that it can be just that. Every victory in Cancerville is huge and beyond description. The good news is that it happens more and more every day. Please allow me to correct myself. That news is not just good, it is great! Hold onto that headline and strive to make it your own.

In Sum

Try to leave the unknown alone for now; none of us can know the future. Right now, this very moment is certain and the rest is unknown—in and out of Cancerville. Assume your loved one will be okay. Believe that the knowledgeable and talented doctors and their medical staff are working and planning on winning, just as you are. Know that hope makes it easier and sometimes even makes it better.

You really don't have the time or energy to waste on the unknown. Right now, you need to begin to understand Cancerville and its land so you can take it on. Toward that end, we move on to accomplish that in Part II.

PART II

Understanding the Land

CHAPTER 5

I will be able to play a difficult hand well.

Making Eye Contact with Cancerville

When you first arrive in Cancerville, a part of you will not want to acknowledge that you are really there. If you are like me, you will probably close your eyes and make believe that you are somewhere else. You may even try to do that with your eyes open. You will likely do your best, especially if you are male, to talk to no one else in Cancerville, pretending you are a visitor rather than a resident.

You may also think, like I did, that it is a case of mistaken identity—not my daughter's turn! Eileen, upon receiving her cancer diagnosis, said, "Are they sure it isn't Sally's or Jane's test results, not that I wish anything bad for them?" Susan was given the results of her CT Scan that diagnosed her cancer in the ER. She reviewed it like the devoted nurse she was, thinking and feeling it was about someone else. Terry knew something was not right in his body, but never imagined he, a rugged Lacrosse player and coach, could have bladder cancer. The immediate need to detach from Cancerville and deny the diagnosis is a very reliable event. Who can really blame people for wanting to believe it is a case of mistaken identity?

For the majority of people, the transition into Cancerville takes time; entering Cancerville is really not unlike any other new and difficult situation. There is a learning curve. There is a time frame within which you will adjust and adapt. Obviously, you will never like Cancerville, but you will figure out how to dislike it less. You will also learn how to manage it better. There is probably no one who can immediately go from the shock of the diagnosis to taking on Cancerville full tilt.

Becoming Empowered in Cancerville

Eventually, you will need to go face-to-face with Cancerville. Doing so is an important part of accepting this most unfortunate reality. Although acceptance may sound completely undesirable right now, acceptance will allow you to move forward and take on Cancerville's challenges. The sooner you make eye contact with Cancerville, the faster you can be present in an empowered way for yourself and an empowering way for your loved one. All of this progress paves the way for you to begin to understand this complicated land and figure out how you can be most helpful to yourself and your loved one.

By going face-to-face and staring down Cancerville, I don't mean to say that you should be glaring at it, flooded with all of your anger and resentments. I am referring, instead, to feeling strong and powerful there, and being able to hold your own. I will grant you that Cancerville creates a bit of a David and Goliath feeling, but just remember who won that battle. Please hold that thought for a moment.

In the beginning, Cancerville is a very intimidating place. Soon it will become a place where you will feel more able to take on its challenges with strength, courage, and determination. The sooner you face Cancerville directly and begin to stare it down, the better you will feel. Your goal is to own this land for the duration. As we continue to walk through Cancerville together, I will help you to do just that.

Being Patient with a Clumsy and Cumbersome Medical System

As you already know, you are entering Cancerville at a very peculiar time in the delivery of medical services in the United States and many other places as well. While the technological side of medicine has never been stronger, the rest of it is in disarray. It is sad to see and say that the entire medical system appears to have lost its way.

One day while visiting Jodi in New York, Ronnie developed strong pains that seemed like those of a heart attack. Given her stress levels at that time, it wouldn't have been surprising if that were the case. So we all jumped in Zev's car, which he drove ambulance-style sans siren (though, come to think of it, he always drives that way) to the ER of St. Vincent's Hospital in the West Village. After several uncomfortable hours of waiting, the doctors told us that Ronnie probably had had a gallbladder attack. It was just another crazy day in Cancerville. Her gallbladder was removed a few months later.

In the October 25, 2010 issue of *New York Magazine*, St. Vincent's Hospital was declared dead on arrival. Better them than my wife the day she went there! The sad news was that St. Vincent's, along with sixteen other hospitals in New York City, had closed since 2000. St. Vincent's, around for 160 years, had treated victims of the Titanic, the Triangle Shirt Waist Factory fire, and 9/11. They had such a strong legacy, but such a weak balance sheet. St. Vincent's was one billion dollars in debt and drowning to the tune of ten million dollars a month. This is just one small example of this strange time in the medical field.

Being Patient with the Process

It is likely that there will be multiple frustrations in Cancerville ranging from lost documents, to mis-scheduled appointments, to hurry-up-and-wait times, to short supplies of medications, to a variety of insurance confusions. Cancerville is often a slow experience that demands a one-day-at-a-time perspective. The picture in your mind before you entered Cancerville may have been that it works with precision and in fast motion. In reality, it can be a drawn out process that moves like a slow golf cart that needs a battery charge. With so much racing through your mind, your frustrations can multiply at each turn, delay, and detour.

If you ever needed patience, you need it now. Know that even when it doesn't seem like it, the medical team is doing their very best. They are lifeguards on a stormy beach. They are focused on the choppy waters and helping the people there get back to shore. The more you can be patient, the more your loved one, the patient, can be as well. Maybe that is where the word originated.

HIPAA Hip, Not Hurray!

What also complicates the present-day medical scene is that it is now driven by the HIPAA privacy act and Risk Management policies. This means that "bureaucrazy" rules in the medical community, and unfortunately, Cancerville is no exception. My goal in sharing all of this information is not to overwhelm you or to worry you in advance, but I have promised to be honest with you. This area of Cancerville is probably best explored sooner rather than later. Clearly, you and your loved one will need to learn how to manage all the paperwork, insurance issues, and bureaucratic obstacles without it getting you down.

So what does all of this mean for you in Cancerville? There will literally be a forest full of trees converted into papers for you to sign. In addition, there will be disclosure statements and releases that sound like they were written by Attila the Hun, Jack the Ripper, and the U.S. Supreme Court.

Please don't go face-to-face or try to stare down these forms. Just have your loved one close his or her eyes and sign them. Your attorney might advise otherwise, but this is my opinion. Ronnie recently had to sign a zillion forms for a simple cataract surgery, and I advised her to do the same. I clearly remember the ones specifically created in Cancerville that Jodi asked me to review. I didn't understand a word of it. I simply encouraged her to sign on the dotted line so she and the process could move forward. Even Rob, an attorney, agreed and did the same with all of the papers related to Jake's treatment.

On Not Displacing Your Angst

Although your nerves are hypersensitive and you may be feeling hyper, try not to let the less important frustrations get to you. It might be helpful to refer back to the relativity chart in Chapter 1 and use it as a guide. Please do your best, as well, to not take your frustrations out on staff members who are really just following standard operating procedures and doing their jobs. None of the people you will interact with created HIPAA or the disclosure/release forms you will be asked to complete. In fact, the staff probably finds them just as annoying as you do. At least you will only have to sign them, while the staff has to sort, staple, and store all those forms appropriately.

Going face-to-face with Cancerville demands patience and courtesy outside the medical arena as well. It is easy to displace all of your angst and frustrations onto the innocent others with whom you interact. For example, I remember speaking rudely to an employee at my gym when he shut the steam room a little earlier than usual one night. This is not my typical style, and after thinking about it, I was sorry for what I had done. The next time I saw him I apologized. I simply shared with him that I was going through a difficult time and didn't mean to take it out on him. Since then we have enjoyed a nice rapport and he seems to go out of his way to be friendly as he checks me in or waves good-bye.

To stare down Cancerville, you need to be comfortably balanced and in charge of yourself. If you have a little slip-up like I did at the gym, make peace and move on. We will talk more about your Cancerville angst and reining in your anger in Chapter 14.

Coping with the Environs of Cancerville

I remember riding the elevator at Sloan-Kettering in July, surrounded by many young, hairless folks who appeared pale and weak. Some were in wheelchairs attached to IV lines; few wore smiles on their faces. That scene was neither calming nor comfortable. In fact, it made me want to break down and cry.

Sadly, the imagery is even more difficult, daunting, and draining in the children's wings of Cancerville. But remember that in the hospitals and medical facilities of Cancerville, you mostly see the people going through treatment at that very moment, rather than seeing all of the survivors who are back to their everyday lives. It can really help to visualize that positive outcome for every person you see going through treatment, as there are millions who have gone through Cancerville and have been cured. The survival rate from cancer overall has almost quadrupled since the late 1970s.

The gray and somber mood of Cancerville sometimes extends to the facilities themselves. Of course, facilities vary widely, but many lack a calming or cheerful ambience or even basic creature comforts. Often, they appear to be cold, even on a hot July day. We decided to take a private room for Jodi's comfort after her surgery. Even so, it was much smaller than we expected. Ronnie stayed with Jodi the three nights she was there and had to sleep on an uncomfortable reclining chair. The out-of-pocket charge for such "luxury" was over five hundred dollars per night—yet the Plaza or Pierre it was not!

In the same vein, Rob felt that the facilities for children at Sloan-Kettering were disappointing, to say the least. Moms slept on recliners and showered in shabby community bathrooms. The playroom for the children was inadequate. According to his son Jake, "Even the bingo prizes sucked." In that family's signature style, they brought in toys and crafts for the other children to enjoy. Jake, in the midst of his own challenges, would make cards for the other children and hand them out daily to cheer them up and wish them well. He also donated all the gifts and money he received from family and friends to the bingo loot bag. The apple does not fall far from the tree!

Clearly, making eye contact with and staring down Cancerville sometimes requires tolerating less than comfortable conditions and making the best of them. It may help to remember that you and your loved one are not visiting Cancerville for the food and facilities. You are there for a cure. That is all you want and all you need. In reality, it is better for the monies to go into research, than into fixing up the place.

You are not being unreasonable if the depressing environs bother you in a cancer facility. Ambience and décor can certainly influence your mood in many positive ways and help lift your Cancerville state of mind. In addition to being there almost 24/7 for the many months he was there, Jake's mom recognized the value of a positive environment for her son and the whole family. She brightly decorated his long-term room at Sloan-Kettering and filled it with warm wall hangings and the ambient equivalent of a happy smile. She changed the decorations weekly and went all out for holidays such as July 4th, Halloween, and Thanksgiving. Now that is what I call taking charge!

Strength comes from making a silk purse out of a sow's ear, as the expression goes. If you have the time, energy, and option of being creative like Cristina, you may want to do what you can to improve the physical environment in Cancerville. This is a small, but significant, example of facing Cancerville head-on and taking charge of what you can. You will feel just a little more powerful and your and your loved one's mood will be lifted as well. If upgrading the ambience is not an option for you, try to focus on your dedicated medical team and their powerful ammunition. Please remember that it is their medical expertise rather than the environs that truly distinguishes Sloan-Kettering and so many other cancer centers.

I learned that Sloan-Kettering holds a prom in June for all of the children and teens who have been there during the year.

There is food, music, dancing, and fun. Cristina, Rob, Jake, Chase, and Phil attended, as did over one hundred patients, family members, and all of the staff, nurses, and doctors. The latter wore tuxes and prom dresses, while providing the same for the children.

Hearing about and picturing this prom brought a few tears to my eyes, as I envisioned the sometimes grim-faced doctors happily dancing with the children whose lives they had saved. Perhaps some of my tears were for Jake having been voted Prom King. Believe me when I say he earned that title in every imaginable, and at times unimaginable, way. Rob nicknamed him "The Warrior" for good reason!

Rob asked Jake if he was surprised when they named him Prom King. His reply tells us what really makes cancer centers special. Jake said, "No, not at all. I knew I was going to win when I heard that the nurses were the ones voting—all my nurses loved me." That illustrates at least two things: first, that this young boy finally got to take charge of Cancerville and stare it down in the sweetest of ways—for one magical night Jake was the King of Cancerville. Second, that a little boy believed so strongly in his nurses' love clearly shows that the human factor is far more important than the facility. I hope all of this helps you believe in the commitment and dedication of cancer center teams all over the world; the expertise and spirit of the medical staff is what really counts. We can cope with the facilities.

Feeling Stronger

Making strong and serious eye contact with Cancerville requires coming at it with resolve. This means confidently knowing that you and your loved one will be able to tolerate everything that comes at you and then some. Resolve also implies your determination to keep bouncing back whenever, if ever, you have a momentary meltdown. Meltdowns tend to go with the territory, so don't be upset with yourself if you have one. These happen to the strongest of us from time to time because Cancerville is one tough trek. Yet I am confident that you can meet Cancerville head-on and hold your own. Use all of the positive stories coming out of there to support your strong approach.

There is one more way in which you can take on Cancerville and try to make it a more level playing field. In private, look in the mirror and make a tough grimacing face like a wrestler or martial artist. Look mean and bare your teeth as if you were about to bite and fight and rip your opponent's head off. Make believe that Cancerville lies beyond the mirror and grunt and growl in a show of power. That's facing Cancerville head-on, staring it down, and hanging tough against a formidable opponent.

Use that strength and draw from it, believing that your loved one will be okay. Keep that in the forefront of your mind as you stare down Cancerville every single day. Aim your slingshot right at its hateful head and assume your loved one, like David, will win his or her battle too.

When I wrote the above, I had no idea that people at Columbia and Harvard Universities were researching postures and the effects of what they termed "embodiment." Their research had people assume either high or low-power poses. An example of the former is someone standing and leaning slightly forward. The latter is someone sitting with hands crossed and head bent slightly down. Harvard and Columbia haven't experimented with my pose of growling into the mirror just yet, but I am confident they will try it soon.

Those who took the stronger power poses had significantly higher post-pose cortisol and testosterone levels (fight hormones) than those who took the more passive positions. This suggests that power posturing promotes the activation of mind and body chemicals that energize our strength. Those inner forces are just what you need to take on and stare down Cancerville. So grunt and growl even louder and show more of your teeth. Embody strength in every way that you can, and the likelihood is, by doing that, you will generate more strength.

I came across another story that suggests that staring Cancerville down can help the patient as well as family members. A *Sun-Sentinel* article titled "ESPN's Scott Fighting His Cancer Head-on" said, "Scott is to journalists what Lance

Armstrong is to athletes. He's fighting and excelling during his battle with this ugly disease.... He is showing the world...that cancer isn't an excuse to stop living. It's even more of a reason to start."

Stuart Scott is a popular and well-spoken ESPN anchor. Three years ago he fought off stomach cancer, but it has returned. How is he facing it this time around? He says to his cancer cells, "Nah, dawg, I'm better. I'm stronger. You're not going to beat me."

Beyond those strong, in your face words, he practices martial arts a few days after his chemo treatments to further kick cancer's butt. He says, "It's just who I am so it's not a matter of being impressive, it's a matter of I'm going to win this and this is how I win. It motivates me to win." He concludes the interview by saying, "You can try, but I'm just gonna come harder than you. I'm gonna come harder than you all day long." In Stuart's strong voice and spirit, let me hear you growl!

In Sum

I am confident that you will be able to figure out how to make eye contact with and stare down Cancerville. Remind yourself that your loved one and you are strong enough to take on its burdens and meet them head-on. Have faith in your medical team and work quickly to establish a partnership, despite the bureaucratic hassles. Reach out to talk to others you meet in Cancerville. You just never know where your next moment of inspiration will come from. Above all else, think strong. Cancerville gives us no choice other than to rise to its challenges each and every time.

As part of taking on Cancerville, let's turn to the important subject of meeting with your loved one's doctors. These meetings can be difficult, but it is part of slowly accepting where you are and learning what lies ahead for your loved one and for you.

CHAPTER 6

The doctors, my loved one, and I are all on the same team.

Meetings with the Dedicated Doctors

As people, we vary in terms of our attention to detail. Some want only a brief overview from the medical team while others expect that every issue be clearly explained. Ronnie's nature is the latter, while I am definitely an "executive summary" type. It may be part of my being from "Mars" and my wife being from "Venus." Or maybe, it's because I am of a personality type that goes for the big picture, while she prefers to know all of the details.

Your personal style will greatly influence how you approach your meetings with the doctors. You will bring your nature to the consultation and treatment rooms of Cancerville. Because that is the case, nothing I say here should be seen as absolute. I greatly respect your right to conduct all aspects of your time in Cancerville as you see fit. What I do hope to offer here is a game plan for these meetings.

Please keep in mind that the dedicated doctors are people—just like you and me. Like us, they vary greatly in style, sense, and sensitivity. Please remember that the Cancerville doctors, no matter their natures, are committed to the very same goals that you have for your loved one. They want cancer to lose and your loved one to win. At the end of the day, that is really all that matters.

Getting Past Difficult Meetings

I remember our family meetings with the doctors in Cancerville all too well. We would wait hours to see the doctor for ten or fifteen minutes. In those moments, Cancerville intimidated me in a way few places have. The physicians were harried, and we, I couldn't help but sense, were annoying. They were in a rush and made that known to us, but we had hours of questions. In fact, we wanted to move into their offices for the duration. For better or worse, many physicians are more interested in treating than greeting or meeting nervous and distraught family members. Both positions make sense depending upon the seat in which one is sitting.

I hope that your medical team brings a friendly and encouraging demeanor along with their technical expertise. If you can't have both, I think you will agree that knowledgeable doctors trump cheerful ones. As you already know, not all doctors are created equal. Some, whose bedside manners leave much to be desired, are nonetheless highly skilled and trustworthy practitioners.

In fairness, a doctor's job—especially in Cancerville—is not easy. Having spent my career as a psychologist trying to help a garden variety of unhappy people, I can only imagine how difficult it is to treat and support patients and their families and friends in Cancerville. By two o'clock in the afternoon, many are probably wondering why they didn't go into dermatology. Yet every cancer doctor I have met has been totally dedicated to fighting cancer and being part of an army of hope.

The doctors stand between your loved one and the difficult treatments. They also have the challenging job of standing in front of and blocking the exit door. They don't want to lose your loved one's fight any more than you do. They are determined to minimize your loved one's pain and suffering while saving his or her life. They are on a most serious search and rescue mission and will do everything they can on your loved one's behalf.

Approaching Medical Meetings with More than a Pad

Depending upon the specifics, you may or may not attend medical meetings with your loved one. If you attend, your adult loved one may prefer that you be a quiet listener or a more verbal participant. If you are dealing with a child or teen, your role in these meetings will be significant.

If you are like Ronnie, you will bring a comprehensive list of questions along with pen and paper to take notes. If you are like me, you will just wing it. However, the danger of my approach is that, just like white-coat blood pressure elevations, there can also be white-coat dementia. Thank goodness both are temporary. It is, however, possible to forget both your questions and the doctors' answers as you sit there in a funky fog.

A tape recorder may help if the doctor is okay with that and you are not the note-taking type. It is also helpful to bring another set of ears to listen, ask questions, and remember what is said. Rob's dad, Phil, attended every medical meeting about his grandson, both to support his family and to be that additional pair of ears.

Practically speaking, it is important to limit your questions to those that are essential and answerable. You don't wait hours to see the doctors because they are playing cards in the rec room. In fact, there is no rec room! They are as overworked as any other doctor in America today. Being respectful of their time may help generate goodwill and avoid creating a situation in which the doctor does not take you or your questions seriously.

Receiving Reassurances in Cancerville

I encourage you to accept that you may not get the complete reassurance you want from the doctors. You want to know that your loved one will be okay, but unfortunately, in Cancerville, assurances are not always available; there are just so many unknowns. Instead, give yourself the answer you crave—like a special gift. Assume that "yes, my loved one will be a survivor."

On the other hand, as Cancerville's successes mount, more doctors are more able to be more optimistic. When my friend Howie was diagnosed with kidney cancer, his doctor told him, "I am going to hurt you to save you, but you will be okay." His doctor delivered on both counts. His painful recovery took quite a while, but he is alive, back at work, and well today—six years later. He had been in that position before, twenty-plus years ago, as a younger man when he had cardiac bypass surgery; and seven years ago he suffered a heart attack. His health has not been his strongest suit, but his strength and survival instincts have. Thank goodness for that.

In 2008, prior to becoming a major league baseball player, Anthony Rizzo, who went to high school not far from my home in Florida, was diagnosed with Hodgkin's lymphoma. In a recent interview, he said that he credits his Boston area doctors for being encouraging:

> They assured me everything was going to be OK and I would beat it, no problem. They told me I would be able to play baseball again and just live a normal life. They gave not only me but my family hope. That's an important part of beating cancer. Maintaining hope.

As if to prove his doctors right, Anthony hit his first home run in the second game he played as a major leaguer. What a difference three years can make. "That ball is going, going, and it's gone!" Rizzo is one of many major league baseball players who have won their battles with cancer.

Perhaps you will receive the reassurance you are seeking, or perhaps you will not. It will depend upon the type and stage of your loved one's cancer, as well as the doctor's nature. Other doctors dealing with Howie or Anthony might not have been so positive. They might have decided to wait and see. Unless you have information to the contrary, I strongly encourage you to assume your loved one will be okay. In Parts III and IV, I will teach you tools that can help you influence your thoughts and expectations.

The Information You Will Most Likely be Given at a Meeting

What information and feedback are your loved one's doctors responsible for providing? Here is a brief overview that you can adapt to your particular situation:

Initial Meeting Post-Diagnosis:

- a summary of the test results and confidence in their accuracy
- the diagnosis based on these results, including type and stage (if known)
- the plan for treating the disease
- a brief overview of the impact of treatment on the patient and how to minimize side effects
- the probable time frame of treatment
- what follow-up testing will be done and when
- whether any genetic testing is suggested to help determine heritable origins (if appropriate)
- when the next meeting will take place

Follow-up Meetings:

- progress and any new findings
- unexpected problems that have arisen
- how patient has tolerated treatment
- any changes in the treatment plan
- what follow-up testing will be done and when
- what is happening next
- when the next meeting will take place

These Meetings are a Pain

One of the most difficult parts of these meetings is having them at all. Part of me sat through each one saying to myself, "What are we doing here?" Another difficult part is listening, sometimes over and over again, to the list of possible negative outcomes of the treatments. This information works against your efforts to be positive. Know that such disclosures and disclaimers represent mandatory risk management and malpractice suit prevention. The medical team is required to disclose the dangers of treatment, just as they are required to have your loved one or you sign all those forms. Tune it out as best you can, and assume that none of the possibilities will happen to your loved one.

Former football great and member of the Dolphin perfect season team of 1972, Jim Mandich recently passed from cancer at age sixty-two. It was reported that he interrupted a nurse who was telling him about the hurtful effects of his medication. He said, "The doctors told me all the good it'll do. I don't need to hear the bad." To his credit, Mandich, known for his partying ways, referred to chemo treatment times as "happy hour." How's that for putting a positive spin on a not so pleasant time?

His story reflects your and your loved one's need to be vigilant in blocking out unhelpful negative news. To be clear, there is an obvious and significant difference between being given helpful versus hurtful information. "If you run a fever of more than 101 degrees post-chemo, you need to call the doctor," is helpful to know. "Unfortunately, you are going to feel awful after this treatment," is upsetting and puts negative expectations in your loved one's mind, which can lead to self-fulfilling prophecies—which often come true. If your loved one is told he or she will be terribly nauseated post-treatment, the odds are that he or she will be more likely to feel that way. Better to not be told anything in advance and just wait and see what happens. This is why I never read the information that comes with a prescription; Ronnie, of course, reads every word!

I spoke in Chapter 1 about our tendency to use healthy denial to avoid worrying about a variety of life threatening events. In your meetings with the doctors you can use that denial to your advantage. For example, one of Jodi's chemo drugs could have caused heart problems, so she had to go for periodic cardiac testing. My initial thought when I learned of that potential side effect was: "Great, my daughter will have a heart condition in addition to cancer. Really terrific!"

I responded to my automatic negativity by saying: "Bull on that! She is young, in great shape, works out regularly, and will be fine. There will be no long-term problems." In fact, that Jodi never developed any heart problems confirmed my optimism. It is very important to catch your mind heading south and redirect it to neutral, if not positive, thoughts. We will discuss this important issue in Chapter 11, "The Power of Positive Self-Talk."

Communicating with the Doctors is Essential

Usually, feedback meetings are scheduled on a regular basis while your loved one goes through treatment and even after it is completed. These may occur more frequently with more complex treatments or when trying to accomplish a specific result. In Rob's case, he and his family met with their team of doctors after each round of chemo. They were struggling to get Jake into remission so that his fraternal twin brother, Chase, could provide his bone marrow, as he was a perfect match. This is why Rob nicknamed Chase "The Hero."

Four grim-faced meetings with the doctors indicated poor chemo results, precluding the possibility of a bone marrow transplant. Rob's emotional knees buckled under the pressure but he rallied back quickly. After the fifth rough round of chemo, the doctors finally achieved their goal, which they announced in a far more upbeat meeting. Their relief, however, was quickly neutralized by the need for another demanding round right before the transplant. The doctors took this boy to the edge of his life in order to save his life. Truth!

I am quite sure that it was not important to Jodi that we be present at all doctor meetings. In fact, my guess is that at least a few times she would have preferred just going to them with Zev. She knew, however, how important it was to us to be there and was kind enough not to exclude us from them. I recall one time when we flew back and forth from Florida in one day just to attend an important meeting and enjoy lunch with our daughter. I am not sure that would be necessary in today's hi-tech world of video conferencing. Then again, my guess is that my wife would still want to be there in person. That's just who she is and how she is wired as a mom.

Between Doctor Meetings

When you are in between doctor meetings in Cancerville, try to assume that no news is good news. Doctors don't pull any punches there. They don't like to report bad news. However, if there are any complications, physicians are ethically and legally bound to share that information with patients and/or their families.

In my opinion, the best thing you can do is to stay out of the way and let the medical team do their job. Wait for them to communicate. They will not leave you out of the equation, as communicating and updating their patients and their families are important parts of their job.

However, I did feel the need to email Jodi's surgeon twice at Sloan-Kettering with a question. Each time it had to do with something I had read in a magazine or newspaper. He was kind enough to respond reassuringly the same day. He was quick to remind me that a magazine is not a scientific journal and that the information didn't apply to Jodi. That kind of response helps one to get back on a positive track quickly. As I have said, when dealing with Cancerville, remaining positive is an on-and-off process. It is easy for even the most optimistic person to be temporarily derailed by someone's comment, a magazine article, or any other information that hits in a sensitive place.

When calling or emailing the doctor, try to use discretion. Sending daily emails or making frequent phone calls will not be appreciated. Instead, pick your queries carefully and remind yourself that the doctor is helping many patients and families all at the same time.

You can fill in some of the blanks by reading relevant books and checking reliable Internet sites for additional information. I read at least six books on breast cancer as well as others, including Lance Armstrong's inspiring account of his experience in Cancerville, *It's Not About the Bike*.[6] Both you and your loved one may find Bernie Siegel's book *How to Live Between Office Visits* very helpful as well.[7]

On Being an Involved Support

There are, however, certain situations that demand your vigilant attention. Ultimately, you and your loved one have the right to question, obtain second opinions, seek out information, or try to change to a different doctor or setting to ensure the care provided is the best available.

I am encouraging you to trust your medical team. I am also, however, acknowledging your and your loved one's right to thoroughly check out and become informed about each phase of treatment. This is especially true if it is not going according to plan. That is why Rob maintained communication with two other cancer centers to confirm that they would be using the same protocol for Jake as Sloan-Ketttering.

Your loved one, the team of doctors, and you are partners in the search for the cure. They will most likely support your desire to get second opinions or go to a place where relevant trials are being conducted, etc. In many instances, they will guide you in those directions. Obviously, if your loved one is a child or teen, he or she is not able to participate in this doctor-patient partnership and you will be the representative.

As far back as 1979, Norman Cousins promoted an informed doctor-patient partnership in his widely acclaimed book, *Anatomy of an Illness as Perceived by the Patient.*[8] He said, "I saw the need to build bridges across the gap that for so long had separated the physician and the public." As those words suggest, all involved individuals need to work together in a collaborative effort. These words are as applicable today as they were back then. They apply as much to Cancerville as they do to any other area of medicine.

Though free to explore all options, nothing I have said is intended for you to encourage your loved one to participate in "fringe" treatments. This is especially true for those approaches that emphasize extreme measures. I would also advise you to be cautious about high-priced, out of the country interventions, helpful as they may sound. My simple-minded belief, with which you may choose to disagree, is that if something were truly a miracle cure, it would be widely and wildly accepted and used everywhere, including America.

Wherever desperate people live, there will be those who try to take advantage of their predicament. Though I encourage your optimism, as you will soon see in Chapter 10, it needs to be realistic and reasonable. I have met several people who chased their loved one's cure all over the world, spent fifty or more thousand dollars, and accomplished nothing. In one situation, a dramatic intervention attempt overseas may have even hastened the patient's passing.

Obviously, whether you are buying a car, moving to a new city, or walking the Cancerville beat, an informed consumer is in a stronger position to adapt, cope, know what to expect, and manage all of the demands. In Cancerville, "consumers" are like tourists in a foreign land. They may have read Frommer's and/or Fodor's books, but will eventually put their trust in a local guide who truly knows the lay of the land. Your local guides in Cancerville are your medical team. They walk the streets day and night. So find a team that you can trust and respect, and allow them to lead your loved one's way back into health.

Watching Out for Sadistic Statistics

Finally, there is a tricky, sticky wicket involved in your quest for information and hopefulness. Cancerville is filled and often flooded with statistics. When they are hopeful and optimistic, we hold onto them with a lover's embrace. When they tilt the other way, we want to burn the book or article or punch the person citing the statistic.

Statistics can be misleading; therefore, you should treat all statistics with a certain level of cautious detachment. They change all the time as new studies and protocols come into being. They are based on large samples and may or may not apply to your loved one's situation; your loved one's circumstance is specific to your loved one. No one statistic, or even a battery of them, will predict your loved one's experience.

I hear of and have met people who were given little chance to survive, but did. Unfortunately, I also know of those for whom Cancerville was supposed to be a slam-dunk and it wasn't. Misleading statistics even apply to the diagnosis itself. Jodi was given a ninety-nine percent probability that her lump was benign. That was reassuring until we learned otherwise. It is best to not get caught up in statistical predictions.

Years ago my doctor friend Bob said, "Bill, in any individual's medical situation, surgery, or disease there is either a one hundred percent chance or a zero percent chance that the person will be okay." In that context, all you can do is assume that for your loved one there is a one hundred percent chance that he or she will be okay and leave it at that.

In *Promise Me*, Nancy Brinker says, "Certainly, a key component to managing one's own cancer treatment or the treatment of a loved one is managing expectations, which means chiseling some kind of reality-based tunnel between statistics and hope." I totally agree and encourage you to give greater weight, whenever it is appropriate, to the hopeful parts.

In Sum

The meetings with your loved one's doctors are not easy, as no one really wants to be there. However, they are an important way to gain perspective about the latest results and the doctors' plans for the future. Cancerville treatment is an ongoing process, as are your communications with the medical team. Sometimes positive results come slowly, and these meetings summarize what has occurred so far as well as the updated plan for the future. Other times, it all falls into place smoothly as treatment proceeds, but even these reassuring meetings are important and helpful.

Approach these meetings with an open mind. Know the doctors on your team want to win just as much as you do. They will do everything in their power to achieve that result. What I said in Chapter 4 about people not liking to lose applies to the doctors as well. They do not want to lose anyone on their "lifeguard" watch.

The physical effects of cancer will be discussed in these medical team meetings. It is essential that you understand and know what to expect, so you can help your loved one deal with these issues. As I reminded myself daily for quite a while, hair does, in fact, grow back! Let's look more closely at this topic in the next chapter.

CHAPTER 7

My loved one's survival is the goal.

Hair Grows Back: Coping with the Physical Effects of Cancer

It is difficult to maintain a positive perspective in Cancerville while observing our loved one's pain and suffering. Let us agree that feeling down, distressed, and disheartened when our loved one is struggling is both appropriate and understandable. I hope the words that follow, as well as those in Parts III and IV, help you cope better during these most upsetting times.

In reality, it is not very complicated. To ultimately help your loved one, the medical soldiers in Cancerville, unfortunately, have to hurt your loved one first. To eliminate cancer cells they often have to use harsh measures. Thus, their arsenal includes administering very strong medications, radiating, operating, and sometimes even amputating. These are all aimed at delivering a knockout punch to those invading cells.

Cancerville treatments are a mean means to a life-saving end. Unfortunately, to kick cancer's butt, the doctors have to kick your loved one's butt too. Because of this, at times, my words won't always help you stay in a positive space. However, because these emotional speed bumps are intermittent, I hope that my words will be helpful and comforting most of the time.

To me, Jodi's hair falling out in clumps, which sadly began the day of her thirty-second birthday, was a visible symbol of all the indignities to which my young and innocent daughter had been subjected since the day she arrived in Cancerville. My friend and colleague Harvey, has a sign in his office that simply says, "No Pain, No Gain." That is the filter through which your loved one's pain and suffering needs to be viewed. That is the way I tried to see Jodi's situation although at times, it was a struggle.

Taking Insurance When the Dealer Has an Ace Showing

As I see it, cancer, I'm sorry and sad to say, is the dealer and always has an ace showing. Your loved one and you have been dealt a poor hand. Therefore, the goal is to outplay the dealer and not to allow him to get blackjack. Your medical team will do all they can to help your loved one and you do just that. Robert Louis Stevenson said it best when he declared, "Life is not so much a matter of holding good cards, but sometimes of playing a poor hand well." That is exactly what we all need to do in Cancerville.

They called Jodi's post-surgical chemo an "insurance policy." I understood what they meant, but hated that she needed it. It implied that, despite her surgery, those sneaky bastard cancer cells could be hiding somewhere within her. It was helpful for me to believe that there were no cancer cells remaining (my healthy denial), but that the insurance was important, nonetheless. I chose to assume that this chemical insurance was not really any different from all of the insurance I have paid for throughout the years, "just in case." You pay the hefty premiums to avoid the risk—Jodi did just that. Your loved one may have to do that, as well, to prevent the dealer from winning.

I had a really hard time watching that liquid insurance flowing through an IV into Jodi's body. I wandered around the hospital in my own self-induced "chemo-brain" dazed state. Ronnie and Zev stayed with Jodi in a small but nicely appointed room, donated by the Lauder family. To both their pride bank credit, and my shame and blame account entry (more about these in Chapter 9), they were able to make small talk and lift her spirit. To my credit, I resisted looking for spirits and gave up any claim to the men's room bar at Sloan-Kettering. Progress in all areas is slow but steady.

Let's be clear that I have been describing Jodi's experience with chemo. There are so many variations when it comes to chemo and other procedural recommendations. In some cases, chemo will occur before additional treatments; in others, it may not be needed at all. For some types of cancer it may be essential, as it was in Jake's case. Fortunately, he also had an ace in his hand. His brother, Chase, was the "Ace" waiting in the wings to save him.

Throughout his blogs, Rob referred to his brave sons as Jake the Snake ("The Warrior") and Chase the Ace ("The Hero"). Jake's Snake nickname was given long before he became ill; Chase's Ace was new, but very much needed to counter the dealer's ace. Together, Chase and Jake got 21. The dealer busted! The good news is that in Cancerville, as this story shows, even though the dealer has an ace showing, the doctors have many of their own and other good hands, including those of the surgeons, to help your loved one.

Striving to Accept Your Loved One's Treatments

It took me quite a while to accept the fact that, if there were any remaining cells, those powerful chemicals were attacking them and insuring my daughter's safety. Thus, if I were thrust back in time into the thick of Cancerville, I would have stayed in that room with Jodi. I would have felt relief instead of grief as every ounce of helpful medication entered her body to kick the sorry little opportunistic asses of the cancer cells.

I would have cheered both the chemo and Jodi on, just as she cheered for her team as a young cheerleader at football games in Coral Springs, Florida: "Two-four-six-eight, what and who do we appreciate—cancer treatments, cancer doctors, nurses, and medical teams. Yeah!" If I knew then what I now feel, I would have focused on the importance of that temporarily disruptive, but life-protecting, liquid.

The short-term side effects of chemo are a consequence of it doing its job. That is what is important to focus on and that is the point I struggled with when we were in the thick of Cancerville. I want to stress, one more time that most side effects are temporary; I don't want you to miss that. I want you to embrace the fact that hair grows back. I remember how excited Jodi was to show Ronnie that she could finally make a very tiny, but for her significant, ponytail. The medicine had destroyed the enemy, but not her hair follicles. Her beautiful long hair grew back, not quickly, but eventually.

You do not have the power to lessen the negative aspects of Cancerville's treatments anymore than you had the power to prevent your loved one from getting cancer. Your power lies in bringing help and hope to the not so nice scenes when they occur.

Sample Words of Support

If a family member or friend of a Cancerville patient and I were talking in my office, here is what it would sound like:

Mom: Bill, I can't take them torturing him. I love him.

Me: I understand. When your loved one is hurting, it rips through you and tears at your heart.

Mom: I can't stop thinking about it. It haunts me day and night.

Me: It would be much better if you could try to stop thinking about it all the time.

Mom: How?

Me: By seeing his pain in a different way. Your son's pain and suffering is not for naught. It is part of fighting his disease and destroying his out-of-control cells. It is a search and rescue mission, even though the search doesn't work as quickly as Google does. It aims at the cancer cells and, unfortunately, hits some of the healthy ones as well. His pains are temporary. Hold onto that thought. Let it play out in your mind for just a moment.

Pause

Mom: Okay, but what about his scars from the surgery?

Me: Scars heal and fade. Even if they don't, they are a small price to pay for winning the Cancerville war.

Mom: But what if he loses the war?

Me: That thought is off the table and needs to be out of your mind or it will drive you out of your mind. I'm going to assume that your son will win. I want you to do that as well.

Mom: It's not easy.

Me: I know. That's why we meet and you read, listen to relaxing music, and do relaxation exercises and yoga.

Mom: Despite all of that, I keep falling off the damn mountain.

Me: Everyone does. What is important is that you always get back up. Feel proud of that.

Mom: I just hate to see him bald. He had such beautiful blond hair.

Me: Hair grows back. His beautiful blond hair will be long and thick again.

Mom: No, he wore it short.

Me: Even better. It will take less time for it to grow back.

Mom: Thank you, Bill, for your support. I always feel better when I leave your office.

Me: You are welcome. See you next week. Call me if you need to. You have my cell number.

Let's Just Move Forward!

Recently, I decided to pay attention to the local newspaper for a few weeks to see what trauma and tragedies were occurring outside of Cancerville. I was, frankly, surprised at the extent of these occurrences. It helped me realize that, unlike headlines that appear after a tragedy occurs, Cancerville often prints its headlines in advance. As soon as you receive the diagnosis, the doom and gloom press releases start forming in your mind. Please try your best not to "write" these as they don't apply right now and, most likely and hopefully, never will.

I read many articles involving unexpected tragedies: a pregnant woman and University of Miami student, both killed while crossing the street in separate accidents; a man sitting on a bus bench being hit by a car and having his arm severed; an eight-year-old dying of Tay-Sachs disease; and a golf course worker who died instantly when he was hit in the head with a ball. These were all sad and shocking stories, but an even more poignant one appeared and appealed to my never-ending belief in people's strength.

A seventeen-year-old girl was heading to class at her high school in Ft. Lauderdale, Florida. A car driven by an older woman suddenly swerved out of control and ran her over. She lived, but lost a leg just above the kneecap. Upon her release from the hospital, she showed maturity, wisdom, and courage not typical of a teen who had just suffered a major functional and narcissistic injury.

At a news conference, she thanked all who helped her, including the medical staff, her family, friends, and others who offered their support. Then she said some of the most incredible words I could ever imagine:

> If I keep working at it and practice, I think I'll get through it....the thought never really occurred to me to, like, wallow in self-pity. I just thought, it's happened. There is nothing I can do. Let's just move forward.

Wow! Couldn't all of us in Cancerville take a lesson from this young woman's accepting and optimistic playbook? As has been said, "The child is the father of the man."

"Let's just move forward!" needs to be a battle cry for all in Cancerville.

In Sum

Hair grows back. Scars heal. Life, hopefully, goes on. Your loved one's pain is difficult to endure, but you will deal with it, and so will your loved one. Time may not heal all wounds, but it does help. Defeating cancer is undeniably the main focus for all of us in Cancerville. Whatever it takes to do that needs to be tolerated and ultimately accepted. Insurance such as Jodi experienced, even though "costly," is a small price to pay for life.

I believe physical scars heal more quickly than emotional ones. As we move on to discussing how to better cope with the emotional effects of cancer, I will help you learn to strengthen your ability to do that. Let's just move forward—slowly, but surely. Using that battle cry will keep your mind stronger in Cancerville.

CHAPTER 8

I will keep my mind strong in Cancerville.

Minds Come Back: Coping with the Emotional Effects of Cancer

Just like hair grows back, minds slowly return close to where they were before your loved one entered Cancerville. It does, however, take a while. Both hair and minds grow slowly. Perhaps it is because they are one above the other. More seriously, it is because Cancerville packs a wallop to both hair follicles and matters of the mind.

Resilient as our minds are, they were never quite built to withstand the ravages of the war on cancer. In fact, minds were not built to withstand war in general. Witness the many soldiers returning from the battlefields of Iraq and Afghanistan who, while not physically injured, have suffered severe emotional upheaval. The number of soldiers affected emotionally grows even higher when we include those who have sustained serious and disabling injuries.

Those actual war zones, as well as that of Cancerville, play out over months and even years of time. This runs contrary to our fast-paced technological lifestyle, which measures experiences in nanoseconds. Most of us don't do very well with slow rides filled with ambiguity and uncertainty, perhaps all the more so because of our modern accelerated sense of time.

Coping with the Unknown

Just about all of us need clarity and closure. No one wants to be haunted by unanswerable questions. Thus, the unknown outcome of Cancerville becomes a torment unto itself. Tell us all will be well and we will walk to Alaska and back barefoot. But tell us to wait and see, and our minds drift toward negative and unacceptable spaces to fill in the blank unknown. It is much better for you to fill in the blanks with strong statements of survival. The more positive you can be in Cancerville, the better you will manage being there.

When I spoke via cell to Susan on her way to Miami to receive the results of her latest CT Scan, she said she was very agitated. "Of course," was my immediate reply, she had every right to be worried. She was about to receive some important news that could make a very big difference in her situation and its outcome.

Minds buckle under that level of anticipatory anxiety. That is okay as long as you don't allow yours to become completely undone. Try to go into every meeting expecting positive news and accepting that if you don't get it this time, you will the next. In this regard, think about Rob and his family's fifth, finally positive meeting with the doctors. The previous four very difficult meetings faded as they slowly, but surely, just moved forward!

Despite my pushing hopeful, positive, and optimistic perspectives, I am neither indifferent nor insensitive to the emotional upheaval that Cancerville causes. I am simply trying to help you offset and counterbalance the negatives when you can.

Cancerville and PTSD

I am convinced that many, if not all, of the patients who go through Cancerville develop a form of Post-Traumatic Stress Disorder (PTSD). I also believe that we in the family and friend position can develop a similar but more limited syndrome by proxy. PTSD usually occurs when someone has a near-death experience from a car or plane accident, fights in a war, or experiences any assault or hostage situation. After writing the above words, I found the following in *Psychiatric Annals,* "Studies have shown cancer treatment can lead to posttraumatic stress disorder-like symptoms." Mortal dangers can create immortal fears.

The symptoms of PTSD, in and out of Cancerville, include depression, anxiety and agitation, difficulty sleeping, nightmares, flashbacks, and other haunting feelings. The person with PTSD has difficulty leaving the traumatic encounter behind. It follows him or her in upending waves that return over and over to the emotions associated with the original experience. It is trauma with a capital T.

This is precisely why I said in the introduction to this book that that very difficult day at Sloan-Kettering would be forever tattooed onto my brain. Though I can help you neutralize and resolve much of the Cancerville emotional residue, there will always be some memories and images that remain with you. I have them and it is likely you will too.

It is clear why this is the case. As people, we do not suffer death potentials gladly or easily; we are programmed for survival. Even when we are not the fittest, we strive to survive and stay alive. Think of Aron Rolston, the man who hacked off his arm so he could free himself from the rocks in which he became stuck while mountain climbing. In 2010, they made a movie, *127 Hours*, about his traumatic, but life-saving, experience.

I want you to try to stay positive and calm, but I am not expecting you to be a robot. We are all sensitive to many issues, especially when it comes to our loved ones. It is likely that, at times, your "stiff upper lip" will quiver and temporarily sag. That is okay as long as you regroup, refresh, and remind yourself that there is a war going on that demands an ongoing fight. In Part IV, I will talk about a variety of tools you can use to help lessen the traumatic impact of Cancerville. For now, let's just understand that it will take a while for your and your loved one's minds to calm and heal from the battles that you face in Cancerville.

The Emotional Effects of Chemo

There is yet another emotional issue with which you will need to deal. Jodi termed it "my chemo brain," and I know that she is not the first or the last to use that term. She used that expression to explain her shifts in mood and attitude that could literally turn, not so much on a dime, but on what seemed like a relatively minor trigger. She could go quickly from fine and calm, to not so fine and not so calm, to very agitated and angry. All of a sudden, and sometimes for no clear reason, Jodi would flood out emotionally. This would cause a commotion of tears, temper, and tirades that were very uncharacteristic of her typically sweet, kind, warm, gentle, and quiet nature.

Clearly, the scenes of Cancerville, comingled with the meds, weakened Jodi's mind and created many emotional ups and downs. I will explain why this occurs in the next chapter. Be alert to this possibility during your loved one's stay in Cancerville; try your best to be a calming influence, rather than buying into the angst and allowing it to escalate. If you struggle with these types of scenes, call Zev. He gets the "patience prize" for getting routinely slammed and not fighting back. His love potion for Jodi was, and is, a salving antidote to the chemo potions that were being pumped into her, as well as all of the trauma she experienced. If you can't reach him, check out Chapter 20, "Communication in Cancerville."

The Spring 2011 issue of *Cure* magazine featured an article titled "Chemo Brain." It spoke about research showing shifts in cognitive functions as a result of chemotherapy. These included memory loss, difficulty retrieving known words, and problems concentrating. People who have undergone chemo have complained about these things for years, and now these studies have begun to validate their frustrating experiences. Perhaps, in the not too distant future, the emotional effects of chemo will also be studied and will confirm what Jodi and many others already know—that harsh medicines affect emotions already sensitized by the demands of the Cancerville experience.

Please keep in mind that you possess some powerful potions of your own that can help with all aspects of chemo brain and really all aspects of Cancerville. These are not complex emotional compounds. For example, a few kind words of support or reassurance, a loving look, or a simple hug all work wonders. These are far more effective than fighting back or saying, "You're crazy, I can't take it anymore," or, "Stop being an idiot." Now is the time to respond with love. Read Bernie Siegel's previously mentioned book, *Love, Medicine and Miracles,* or any other that helps guide you through this land-mined area.

The Resilience of Our Minds

My belief in the potential of minds to bounce back is not based on wishful thinking or idle chatter. It is based on observing the human mind up close and personal for more than forty years. It is based on sitting with thousands of people wounded on the battlefields of life. Some were in Cancerville, while others were in Anxietyville, Depressionville, Divorceville, or some other not so great place.

The majority of these people, especially those who made a serious commitment to themselves, healed and moved forward. In most cases, their experience, painful as it might have been, helped them to grow. From their pain came real and long-lasting gain. The same can, and hopefully will, be true for you and your loved one.

I have always believed that as a therapist I have helped facilitate personal growth, but that the person I was helping did most of the work. Although we all have our breaking points, people eventually can and do bounce back. They may not do this with the force and speed of a bungy cord, but in their own time and way, most people rebound. I am pleased to share that eventually our family did. As part of our healing, we rediscovered some important life lessons, which will be discussed in Chapter 22.

In Sum

The emotional demands of Cancerville lessen over time and resolve themselves. Our loved ones and we ultimately adapt to the changes that occur. This is no different from the high school girl who lost a limb when hit by a car but who has moved on. She returned to school just thirty-two days after the automobile accident that traumatically changed her life forever. This accident may have taken half her leg, but it did not take away even half an ounce of her spirit. Perhaps it even spurred her on. I expect to hear great things about her in the future. Her strength, courage, and optimism can inspire us all.

The same needs to be the case for you and your loved one. Life is always about accepting and adapting to change because no one lives a static existence. "Life," as someone said to me yesterday, "is not always perfect. We make the best and do our best." We were built to be flexible. In Cancerville, perhaps to your surprise or wonderment, you will see that you and your loved one are able to accept, adapt, and cope, even better than you might have expected when all this began.

This suggests that we need to better understand how our minds work and what helps them to work even better. This is a subject that I know like the back of my mind—even more clearly than that. In the next chapter, allow me to share with you how I came to understand how minds work. It is a very interesting but difficult story for me to tell. I suddenly came to learn that my doctoral degree did not come with a vaccine!

PART III

Making the Land Your Own

CHAPTER 9

I aim to be "Dam Strong!" at all times.

How Minds Work

The more clearly you understand how your mind works, the better able you will be to protect it in Cancerville. During my very serious emotional down many, many years ago, I came to understand the workings of my mind and what caused it to not be working so well. I realized this discovery applied to other people as well. I have used this way of describing minds in my work helping others ever since. Hopefully, you will find it useful in keeping your mind as strong as possible, not only in Cancerville, but throughout your life.

Come back with me to 1973. Much of the world was simpler then than now; no Internet, tweets, cell phones, or digital cameras existed. An apple was what you ate to keep the doctor away. The world didn't seem so money focused and neighbors actually talked to each other. That was the year after Ronnie, our two young sons, and I moved to Ft. Lauderdale, Florida. Now that I think about it, our first neighbors were anti-Semitic and didn't allow their children to play with ours. So maybe I'm glorifying things back then just a bit.

Overall, however, it was a user-friendlier world. In spite of that, it was also the year of my serious emotional down. Unfortunately, as I previously said, my psychology degree did not come with a vaccine. All of a sudden I went from calm, cool, collected, and confident to being flooded with overwhelming anxiety. I was wrestling with panic disorder and agoraphobia, but since it was 1973, these words had yet to become part of anyone's vocabulary.

I was diagnosed instead with neurasthenia, a Freudian term that has long since been removed from the *Diagnostic and Statistical Manual* that is used by today's mental health practitioners. Frankly, I still don't fully understand what Freud meant by that diagnosis. To deal with this emotional down, I reluctantly began psychoanalysis once again.

My Struggles with Siggie

My first experience with Dr. Sigmund Freud's ideology occurred in 1971. I was working as an organizational psychologist for IBM in Westchester County, New York, and attending a Freudian postgraduate psychoanalytic training institute at night in Manhattan.

One of the school's self-serving rules was that students had to engage in psychoanalysis with one of their professors. I chose to see and work with a stereotypical analyst complete with an accent and goatee. He began our "work" together by ripping me apart and then set about to put me back together, Humpty Dumpty style. But there was nothing much wrong with me at the time because I wasn't there due to a problem. I was there simply because of the requirement for us to personally experience psychoanalysis. Eventually, I dropped out of Analysis 101 as I realized that my professor's wild interpretations were akin to mental abuse.

Paradoxically, there I was, back on the couch again in 1973 three mornings a week, reviewing every emotional "dirty diaper" of my life. I desperately hoped that it would relieve my constant anxiety. From my analyst's office, I went to mine to help other people with similar problems. Unfortunately, I struggled throughout the day with high levels of physical and emotional discomfort. I helped the people who visited my office a lot more quickly than my analyst and I were helping me.

Five years later, I emerged from that "couch potato" cocoon pretty well healed. In today's world, my colleagues or I could help someone with similar problems resolve them in once-weekly visits within five to six months, rather than years. We have come a long way in helping people with emotional issues by using much more practical cognitive tools and, when appropriate, modern medications. Cancerville has come a long way, as well, in being able to save people's lives. For all the ills of our twenty-first century, it is hard to deny the progress that has been made in just about every life zone.

A Graphic Model of the Mind

While I was trapped in what I came to call Anxietyville, I searched for an explanation of what I was experiencing. I looked through every book I came across, but found none that explained my anxieties. There was nothing back then to help me understand what the people I was trying to help and I were going through. It was the dark ages of mental health knowledge.

I needed and finally found a way to explain myself to myself and help others more clearly understand the basis for their distress. It was a simple, graphic model that described the architecture of the mind. It provided a blueprint to help visualize and understand how minds work. I feel confident this model will teach and encourage you to build a stronger and more protective emotional fortress. It will also help you realize how the mind-strengthening tools I talk about later work and can make an important difference for you and your loved one.

The Importance of Our History

During what I came to call my emotional down, my shrink and I concluded that historical happenings strongly contributed to my hysterical experiences. I also observed that the same was happening with the people I was helping in my office. Hard as it was to understand, old emotional news as far back as the 1940's was making painful headlines in the 1970's.

I give Freud all the credit in this area. He discovered and uncovered the unconscious (subconscious) part of our minds that stores our histories, even if we can't consciously remember all the details. In many ways, he demonstrated how our unconscious both influences and, at times, distorts our day-to-day lives.

My emotional down and all my needless anxiety led me to realize that, in some neurological form, the many neurons and other "wires" in our brains are constantly storing information much like a computer. We all have a "save button" inside our heads. Even if we don't remember the details of what is stored or remember to press save, it happens automatically.

My unconscious was spilling all over my head with the force of a broken water main. Old lessons learned were mixing with new experiences. The "little boy" in me was freaking out about the decisions my adult self had made. My entire being overreacted and felt at risk for disaster. I was a "dam" mess.

The good news is that we can debug much of our early programming and bring those "headlines" up to date. The really neat thing is that we no longer need to clean every emotional "dirty diaper" over years of therapy time. We can now accomplish that much more quickly by using a variety of cognitive and coaching tools.

Initially, it is not easy to understand how our history can cause us emotional difficulties in the present. It seems almost ridiculous to think that what my parents did or said when I was younger could affect what I thought, felt, or did when I was older. However, strange as that may seem to you, it is exactly how our emotional system works. As I said in *Getting Back Up From an Emotional Down*,[9] "Artists in their own unique way, our parents take the clay of our soft, impressionable minds, add some personal colorings, pour us into societal molds, and sculpt us into our personhood." Please know that it is not just our parents that leave their mark. All of our early experiences, our successes and our failures, as well as the influential people we met along the way, affect us in both positive and negative ways.

A Storage Space for Pain

To keep things simple, I suggested that we all have two major storage areas and two additional ones that feed into them. The first stores the hurts and corresponding feelings that we encounter during our journey from birth on through our years of experience. I came to realize that we all have the neurological equivalent of what I called a cesspool, located in the back of our heads.

Our cesspool stores all of the not so pleasant experiences and associated emotions. This includes times we felt or were provoked to feel sad, bad, mad, lesser than, worthless, a failure, stupid, guilty, etc. All of these less than glorious moments are stored in our cesspools. In addition, more serious trauma that includes the death of a loved one; the divorce of our parents; physical, emotional, or sexual abuse; and other difficult and damaging experiences end up occupying large spaces in our cesspools. Please understand that this is not only about our childhood. The pool is always being added to by new cess—our whole lives.

Believe me when I say you would not want to swim in your cesspool; it is, quite likely, polluted. Yet, in some ways, we can sometimes end up doing just that. It is what I was doing in 1973 and for several years thereafter. I wasn't exactly swimming—I was drowning and holding on to my "dam" raft for dear life.

Dam It!

If all we had in our heads was a cesspool, we would all live in a collective state mental hospital where we wouldn't be able to tell the difference between the patients and the doctors. Fortunately, there is another storage center that holds all of our positive experiences. I called that area the dam. This too is built over the course of our entire lives. It is possible to start with a weak dam and build it into a strong one; the opposite is also true.

In that dam of support and protection are our memories of all of the times we felt and were encouraged to feel proud, accomplished, successful, worthy, loved, and deserving. Our dam stores all of the positive, pleasant, and prideful words and images of the good times we have experienced and enjoyed. A strong and solid dam is able to prevent the cess in your pool from flooding over or through it. A person with a strong dam has high levels of self-confidence, self-esteem, and hopeful optimism that help block the cess. These qualities are needed to help you navigate your life in general, and most especially in Cancerville.

A Balance of Powers

In a nutshell, and a very nutty shell at that, we feel and function just fine as long as our dams are strong enough to contain the cess. In contrast, when our dams are weakened, we end up feeling anxious, depressed, distressed, and uncomfortable. This is due to internal or external forces that allow cess to leak through our dams onto our day-to-day functioning. When we go through an emotional down, our dams are as underwater as many mortgages these days.

What inner forces might push our dams down below the water line of our cess? Fatigue, a cold or illness, hormonal shifts, alcohol or drugs, too much sugar, or a variety of other physical events all can weaken dams and diminish our ability to cope. Or, it can occur because cess in our pools is agitated and comes at the inner walls of our dams with the fury and vengeance of a tsunami. In both cases, cess leaks through the dam and causes discomfort in our everyday life.

All kinds of upsetting events can diminish and weaken our dams. Getting in trouble at work can trigger it; losing an important sale can too. Bankruptcy takes us there quickly, as can being caught misbehaving by our spouse. There are, unfortunately, numerous situations and circumstances that add cess to our pools; this in turn agitates us in ways that feel awful and interfere with our comfortable and effective functioning.

Certainly, having a loved one in Cancerville automatically agitates and accelerates cess while weakening your dam. That is precisely why just about every encouragement I offer is intended to help you vent cess and shore up your dam in Cancerville.

Hope, in all of its many forms, supports your dam, while pessimism weakens and puts holes in it, adding to your cess. The following is an illustration of what my mind looked like the day we received Jodi's call telling us that we were all about to enter Cancerville. Obviously, I had some "dam" work to do because my cesspool was flooding through my dam and onto my everyday life.

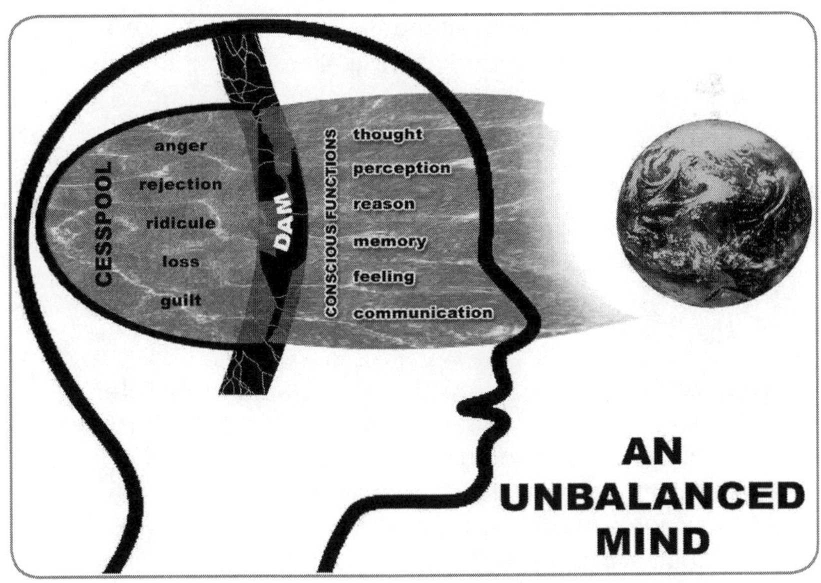

Two Additional Storage Areas

In addition to the cesspool and dam, my belief is that we have two emotional "accounts" that keep track of the cess and dam deposits that we encounter. These are our pride banks and our shame and blame accounts. When we do positive things, it adds to our pride banks, which also contributes to strengthening our dams. When we do things that we later regret, it feeds into our shame and blame accounts, which ultimately end up in our cesspools.

Taking charge of these two zones is important, especially in Cancerville. Your goal is to add consistently to your pride bank and avoid additions to your shame and blame account. Lots of visible VIPs have yet to figure this out. I hope you do. It forms such a simple charter by which to live your life and helps you to make healthy, appropriate, and self-fulfilling choices. Upon reflection, finding the bar in the men's room at Sloan-Kettering was not a great idea. Not only did alcohol feed my depression and anxiety, but it also fed my shame and blame account at the very time I needed to be feeding and filling my pride bank.

One of your many challenges in Cancerville will be to strengthen your dam by adding to your pride bank while minimizing shame and blame entries that add to your cesspool. Unfortunately, the opposite often occurs under stressful and cessful conditions. Stress can bring out your "wild child" in ways that add to your shame and blame account, thereby creating even more cess in a very vicious cycle kind of way.

Stop the Glop

The word I use for that which attracts us to self-defeating shame and blame behaviors is glop. I chose that word to discourage people from indulging; who of us wants to do glop? There is glop in alcohol, nicotine, pill bottles, street drugs, casinos, bedrooms, and even boardrooms, not to mention unhealthy foods that we eat. Glop surrounds us and calls out our name. It tempts us into self-defeating zones and is one of the most destructive forces known to humankind.

We repeatedly see it bring down the strongest, mightiest, and most successful people, as well as those who sit in the opposite position. Obviously, it is much better to go to the gym, a yoga class, or watch a funny movie while we are in Cancerville, than to get drunk, do drugs, gamble, visit porn sites, or otherwise pursue glopful activities. These hurtful behaviors are all part of what I call our "little boy" or "little girl" choices, while the former are healthy adult choices. We all drag our child/teen parts silently behind us via our cesspools, and they can jump out at any moment and make a mess of things. They operate on impulses that seek immediate satisfaction and reflect the poor judgment and risk taking of our younger ages and stages.

I encourage you to do your best to keep your "child parts" in check and stay in your adult zone in Cancerville. Wanting to throw caution to the wind is a tempting but undesirable choice. All of your energies need to be divided between keeping your dam and your loved one's dam as strong and solid as possible.

Cesspools and Dams in Cancerville

Cancerville is a factory that spews out cess, like pollution from an under-regulated industrial plant. I don't have to spell it out for you, as I'm sure you already know what I mean. So much of our added cess and weakened dams in Cancerville are based upon feeling a lack of control, fearing the unknown, thinking about dire possibilities for those we love, and trying to overcome the stresses of a place that is neither kind nor user-friendly.

Even before Cancerville comes along, there is a deep, dark, and scary cave that contains our innermost fears for ourselves and our loved ones. Cancerville inhabits that cave like a large, ferocious, and hungry bear. All of this combines with our old cess to make a strong and forceful partnership of hurtful, disconcerting, and terrifying emotions. This book is a counterforce to scare off the bear. If all else fails, throw it at him!

More Than a Peek into My Pool

I want to use myself as an example to show how cess weakens our dams in general, and particularly in Cancerville. Obviously, our vulnerabilities begin before Cancerville and escalate the day we arrive there. Though I am not a psychologist who tries to needlessly blame parents and other important people in our early lives, there is no denying that they program us in both functional and dysfunctional ways. I owe both my stunning successes, as well as my dismal failures, to my parents, other family members, teachers, and friends. It is likely that you do too.

My anxiety in the 1970's was, in part, related to my very nervous and highly overprotective parents who, unwittingly, taught me that the world was a very dangerous place. My analyst dubbed me "the egg" early on because they raised me to feel as if I was fragile and could easily break. In fact, I did at age thirty, and neither all the King's horsemen nor my psychoanalyst could put me back together again for some time.

In my analysis, however, I discovered many examples of my being programmed by my folks to see the world as a scary place. To learn more about my experiences and find a more complete description of my model of the mind, see my book, *Getting Back Up From an Emotional Down*.

My father's fears were programmed in at sixteen, in 1926, when his father died of leukemia. This sent a clear message to Dad about just how dangerous the world could be. He was forced to leave school and find a job to support his mother and three sisters—he was Cinderfella! From his loss and all those feelings and responsibilities, all the more overwhelming because he was only a teen, came his fears and strong need to feel in control. His worries were palpable and hardly hidden from my view. I learned these "life is dangerous" lessons early, repetitiously, and well. I was an excellent student when it came to "home" schooling. These were all validated when he had a heart attack and died at a young age when I was only eighteen.

By then, my fears were firmly planted within me like weeds, waiting to grow and go wild at age thirty. My emotional down was inevitable. The brilliant psychiatrist, Theodore Isaac Rubin, said in his book, *Compassion and Self-Hate*,[10] "We are all the victims of victims of victims...." In this sense, Dad was a victim of his "scenes and genes." He, in turn, passed that along to me and I, unintentionally, passed the genes along to my sons and the scenes to all three of my children. It is important to note that they and I have successfully overcome these challenges. Hopefully, the muck stopped here!

Much more of my cess came from many loved ones dying young. From my vantage point, death was inevitably linked to youth. It certainly didn't help that I was named for my father's father, a man I never met, but whose grave I was forced to visit every year from a fairly young age. I can still remember staring at my name on his headstone as my father cried for a very long time. In so many different ways, I was taught that we all live on a very precarious perch—every day of our lives!

These experiences explain why I tape-recorded my eulogy on my thirty-fifth birthday in 1977. Can you believe that? It is, strange to say, a fact—in some way, it gave me a sense of control. Yet to do that underscored how convinced I was that I was not long for this world; no wonder I was flooded with anxiety. Perhaps it is significant that many years ago I misplaced the tape containing my eulogy. I am pleased to say that on my next birthday I will be seventy years young!

The combination and culmination of all that cess sitting in my pool from my childhood left me vulnerable to an emotional down. Leaving a stable job and a safe and secure "perch" in New York and moving to Florida, for what quickly turned into unemployment, shouted danger to my "little boy" self, like an alarm going off in the middle of the night. I was now sitting and swaying on that very precarious "perch" I was taught to fear. My cesspool erupted like a volcano in Iceland.

Let's take it one step further to the year 2005 and my arrival into Cancerville. Might my less-than-positive initial entry into Cancerville have been influenced by my parents' teachings all those years ago, so many young people dying among my family and friends, and my emotional down in 1973? Could there have been a direct relationship? I certainly believe there was, but then again, I am one of those "shrink" types. Feel free to disagree if you have a clearer explanation.

My honest sharing of so many people in my family dying young is intended to help you know what is in my cesspool. Please do not allow that to raise your spotlight on catastrophe for your loved one. Many of these people died of causes other than cancer; these ranged from suicide to heart disease. In all cases, in and out of Cancerville, it is likely that these people would have lived if the recent advances in medical knowledge and treatments existed at that time. In a paradoxical way, that can increase rather than decrease our optimism in today's modern medical world.

I hope this description and explanation of how minds work helps yours to work well, even in Cancerville. The formula for that is straightforward—dump your cess, strengthen your dam, fill your pride bank every day, and avoid glop and the shame and blame entries it brings with it. Unfortunately, that is all easier said than done, which is why this isn't the last chapter of my book. I will explain more about how to accomplish all of this as we go along.

In reference to "easier said than done," let's not forget about the glopful bar this most intelligent and aware person found at Sloan-Kettering shortly after entering Cancerville. By working on dumping cess and adding pride bank deposits to strengthen my dam, I was able to lose that bar the same way I lost the tape of my eulogy. It takes time, patience, support, and effort to get back into balance, but I am confident that if you need to, you will. The following is the picture of my mind in Cancerville once I took charge of it and made the land my own. As you can see, my cess was contained by my strengthened dam and was no longer leaking onto the rest of my life.

I aim to be "Dam Strong!" at all times.

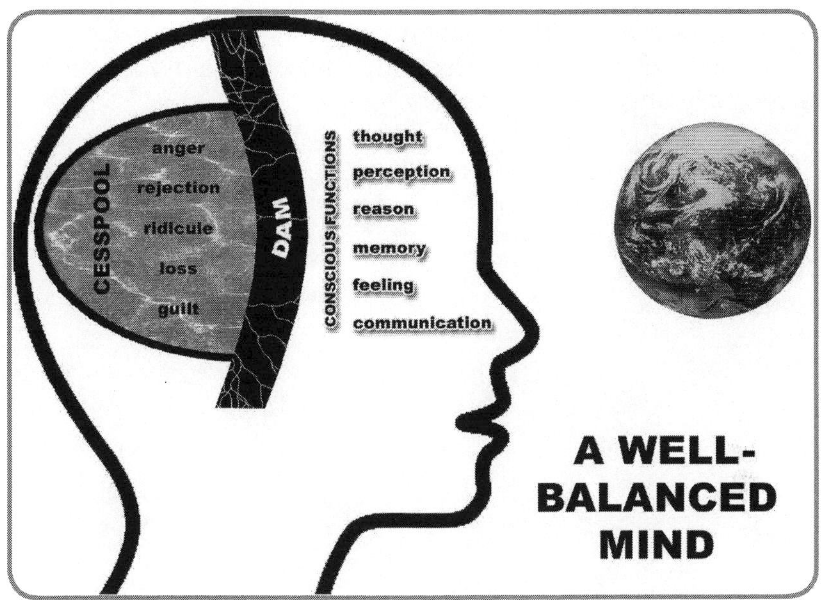

In Sum

I am excited that you can now speak my language. Hopefully, by understanding cesspools, dams, pride banks, shame and blame accounts, and glop, you and I have a whole new vocabulary with which to communicate. You now have a new set of ideas in your dam with which to evaluate your present choices and behaviors. I hope these contribute to your understanding of how minds work and what enables them to work better.

Use these ideas to navigate through the cess-filled streets of Cancerville, while protecting your dam at all times. These simple ideas can help you better understand yourself and guide you to work on areas where your cess is strong and your dam has some cracks and crevices. This visual model of the mind can help you more clearly understand the value of counseling. We will discuss this in more detail in Chapter 17.

Now, as a way to keep your dam as strong as possible, let's take a look at a simple philosophy that can help you remain realistically optimistic in Cancerville.

CHAPTER 10

I will continue to strive for optimism and hope.

Embracing a Really Simple Philosophy: Realistic Optimism

It is not easy, either in life or in Cancerville, to go forward with hopeful and optimistic feelings when they collide with difficult realities. Though our goal is to be strong and positive, the diagnosis of cancer and all that goes with it can rapidly sink our dam, flood us out, and knock the wind right out of our emotional "sails." I remember it all too well.

These choppy, cess-filled waters can throw us right off the boat without a life preserver or raft. Prepare to hold tight to the side of the rocking boat when necessary. My encouragement and plea is that whenever you can, reach out and hold onto a buoy of optimism. I am trying my best to move many of those in your direction.

Research consistently shows that positive mindsets pay multiple dividends in just about all areas of our lives. In Cancerville, we absolutely need that perspective to help get us through. We will discuss this in more depth in the following chapter, "The Power of Positive Self-Talk."

My Evolving Philosophy

When the U.S. economy tanked and people panicked a few years ago, I began to write a blog at *copewiththeeconomy.com*. My goal was to help people stay upbeat and cope better with their financial stresses. Those blogs still exist, as does the other blog it birthed, *mindlymatters.com*. The latter is still being updated every business day to help people deal more positively with all of the stresses in their lives.

I named the philosophy underlying my brief comments in both blogs Realistic Optimism. It encourages a strong, hopeful set of beliefs in line with and tempered by reality. After my Cancerville experience, I came to feel we needed a philosophy that was shaded by neither rose-colored glasses nor black ones. The lenses through which we look at Cancerville and our loved one need to be clear.

My philosophy encourages us to use the clear lens of reality to assess any situation and, where appropriate, add a filter of optimism. For example, in my day-to-day life, reality says that the odds of me winning the Powerball lottery are slim to none. To be optimistic here would be silly, although I might wager a few dollars with the thought that someone has to eventually win. I would not, however, give up my day job before the results were posted. Frankly, I doubt I would give up my day job completely in the unlikely event that I won, as I really enjoy helping people. It fills my pride bank, even if the lottery eliminated my need for piggy bank deposits.

Similarly, in the popular book *The Secret*,[11] which emphasizes the importance of positive thinking, readers are encouraged to visualize checks arriving instead of bills as they walk to their mailboxes. Since there is no connection between people's thoughts and the envelopes the U.S. Postal Service delivers, this seems to be an inappropriate application of positive thinking. Reality needs to be the basis for our optimism.

On the other hand, to be optimistic that I will drive from my home to my office without getting into a car accident would be realistic based on my past experience. That still won't keep me from being realistically vigilant, especially given the drivers in South Florida. The same applies to many potentially dangerous situations that we comfortably approach vigilantly, but optimistically.

Applying Realistic Optimism to Your Cancerville Experience

In Cancerville, this philosophy encourages you to be optimistic within the realistic circumstances of your loved one's specific situation. If treatments are proceeding on course and your loved one is rebounding with resilience, the more optimism you can generate, the better you will feel.

On the other hand, when Jake's situation was not looking promising after four serious post-chemo meetings with the doctors, I encouraged Rob to try to envision the Cancerville equivalent of a Hail Mary pass. I don't think he liked how desperate that phrase sounded, but the truth is that's exactly what happened in that fifth round of chemo. Had I just said to him, "Your son will be fine, so stay optimistic," it would not have been consistent with the reality of that scary time. My credibility as a guide would have been seriously diminished.

Try to stay in the hopeful, positive, optimistic zone until and unless there is clear information to the contrary. Unfortunately, sometimes the reality of the circumstances, right from the beginning, imposes a realistic limit on one's ability to be optimistic.

My seventy-nine-year-old cousin Marilyn was diagnosed with Stage IV lung cancer several years ago and was only given weeks to live. I would not have encouraged her husband or children along the lines of optimism and would not have given them this book to read.

However, if they had called me, I might have encouraged them to hope and/or pray for a miracle. Unfortunately, lotto-like odds limited Marilyn's prognosis from having a happy ending. It was possible she could have beaten them, but not likely. That is where the reality of the situation needs to be considered. Sadly, she died in three weeks.

Yet I recently heard about a woman with the same disease who lived after participating in a clinical trial of an experimental medication; she was the only one of three hundred to survive. Sometimes miracles do happen, just like the story of my friend Tom, whom I previously mentioned.

Good Vibes Going Viral

Not knowing what will happen brings out the frightened, confused, and overwhelmed parts of us in all life's areas, and especially in Cancerville. The philosophy of Realistic Optimism seeks to offset our automatic pessimistic reactions. It strives to replace hopelessness with hopefulness within realistic boundaries. Hope is the cornerstone of life. It is the energy that pushes us to set and achieve our goals, which keep us moving forward instead of standing still or going backward. Hope also enables us to encounter difficult realities and believe that we can overcome them. In my opinion, nothing of significance has been accomplished without hope and optimism.

By empowering yourself in an optimistic direction, you will also empower your loved one. What I have learned from talking to many family members and friends in Cancerville is that their positivism spreads to their loved one and vice versa. Feeling hopeful and optimistic is infectious in a really good way. Hope and optimism spread virally like an interesting YouTube video. You can experience a supportive cycle instead of a vicious one.

As positive feelings bounce back and forth like a colorful beach ball, good vibrations linger in the air and feed your and your loved one's dam.

When you and your loved one are in Cancerville, it is important for you to seek optimism and hope to counterbalance any negativity within you that may arise. The following ideas underscore why that is true:

- There are millions of cancer survivors. Assume that your loved one will be among that group of very strong and special people.
- When you are fighting in any war zone, especially Cancerville, you need to believe your loved one will ultimately win.
- You need to be there for your loved one in both a positive and proactive way.
- You need to maintain your physical and emotional well being because you don't have the time to get sick. In addition, your loved one's immune system may be compromised. Research shows that positivism boosts immune systems.
- Hope is like a flashlight in the dark. In Cancerville, it makes your journey a little easier, helps you find your way, and lightens your load.
- Hope and optimism are assumptions you can choose to make. Take a leap of faith that your loved one will ultimately be okay.

Using Realistic Optimism When Talking with Your Loved One

By promoting optimism and positivism, I am not encouraging family or friends to pretend, blow smoke, or hide concerns from a loved one. Authentic communication resonates better than pretense with the patient. Loved ones become annoyed and/or concerned if they are superficially given feedback that doesn't seem to fit.

At the time I was writing this chapter Susan gave me a relevant article. Last night I read it and discovered that it was very much related to this issue of balance between optimism and realism. Sometimes serendipity seems like more than just coincidence.

The article from *Cure* magazine's 2010 Cancer Resource Guide discusses "protective buffering," a term created by James Coyne, Ph.D. He uses this to describe family and friends suppressing their true feelings to avoid hurting their loved ones. The same applies to the loved one's buffering their complaints to protect their family and friends. As is often the case, professionals are divided about whether this buffering should be done or not. Clearly, without knowing the details, it is hard to say; as in most complex areas, I believe there is a need for balance.

Somewhere between total denial and total disclosure, there exists a reasonable, responsible, and honest way to communicate. Saying that "everything will be fine" or that "everyone survives these days" would be taking optimism to a higher level than I am encouraging. At this too-positive extreme, I have met people whose family members told them that they did not have cancer, even after the medical diagnosis had already been confirmed. Remember that your dialogue and your optimism always need to be based in reality; denying that reality will not help the situation.

Here are some examples of ways to talk to your adult loved one that are realistically optimistic:

- I hate us being in Cancerville, but I choose to believe that this will be okay. We are a strong team and will get through this together. How are you dealing with all of this?
- We will get through this together. I believe you will be okay. Let's pray every day that this will happen. What are you thinking and feeling these days?
- Cancerville is a scary place, but we have a good medical team working to get you well, and I am assuming that that is exactly what will happen. I hope you can embrace

that belief as well, since it really does us no good, and much harm, to be consumed by fear and worry. How is it going on your end?

- I am so sorry to hear about your diagnosis. I am praying for you. How are you dealing with this news? I brought you a book that looks helpful.

These statements, expressions of feelings, and gentle inquiries seem to fall somewhere between saying too little and saying too much. By not buffering your communication with your loved one, you are modeling and encouraging him or her to be more forthright too. How we communicate with children, obviously, will depend on their age. Total honesty may not always fit with children and teens, but positive and reassuring statements are essential.

The Ups and Downs of Cancerville

Reality in Cancerville plays with your mind while it tugs at your heart. Your loved one's slightest ache or pain can rapidly take everyone down dark and dreary paths. Try to bring a flashlight of hope with you during these emotional jogs. Most of the time these speed bumps in your loved one's journey are the equivalent of static on a radio and have no significance whatsoever. Yet, when we are on red alert, every little "noise" becomes an alarm. I do not expect you or your loved one to stay optimistic consistently, but I do encourage you to keep climbing back onto a horse named "Hope" whenever you fall off.

I personally experienced tumbles in Cancerville as my mind and body fell off the "Hope" horse. I scrambled back to get atop "Hope" as quickly as I could. I liked the stride and the strength with which she moved us forward. Let's not forget that rallying cry taught to us by the teen girl who lost a major part of her leg in a car accident—"Let's just move forward!"

Realistically, you will have ups and downs in Cancerville; they come with the territory. It is likely you will have your own personal tumbles as your cesspool overflows in response to someone's comment, a newspaper article, or whatever. Then there will be times when your cess is tripped by your loved one's state of mind and body. Both in and out of Cancerville, when your loved one suffers, you do too. The sooner you get back up on "Hope," if that is realistic, the better you will feel.

In Sum

What I would like you to take away from this chapter is that you can and need to be optimistic and hopeful while facing Cancerville head-on. It is important that your optimism be based on the reality of the circumstances.

I hope you will work to embrace realistic optimism whenever you can. It will make your journey a little easier and be helpful to your loved one as well. Try your best to remain seated and balanced on the horse named "Hope" for as much of your journey as possible. The tools and discussions in the remaining chapters will help you to accomplish that.

Let's move on to discuss positive self-talk. This will give you a voice through which realistic optimism can be achieved. As you will see, I wrote it "dam" strong so you can learn to speak to yourself in an empowering way.

CHAPTER 11

I can write my inner script to be more positive.

The Power of Positive Self-Talk

As you are aware, the words you use to talk to yourself can have a very powerful influence on your feelings, behaviors, and outcomes in a variety of situations. Specifically, the words that form your inner dialogues can take you to dark spaces or, preferably, help you follow the realistic optimism philosophy. This will help you to sustain a more positive outlook in Cancerville.

When I was a boy growing up in the Bronx, there were a couple of people who lived in my apartment building who walked along talking to themselves. We were taught to see them as strange but harmless. At that time, I didn't realize that we all talk to ourselves throughout our waking hours. Now, I know that the difference is that we make sure that our inner chatter and self-talk is silent. This keeps the rest of the world from knowing that we are talking to ourselves.

The Power of Words

As a therapist, I have always marveled at the power of words. Words are the only tools that my colleagues and I have to positively influence the people we help. That we are able to do that for the majority of those who visit us demonstrates just how powerful words—theirs and ours—can be.

A man came into my office today for the first time. He was quite depressed for a variety of rational reasons. He left one hour later with a smile on his face. Did I cure him? Of course not! But I planted some helpful seeds, via my words, which will move him forward over the course of our next several meetings. Because of the advances made in my field, this is a whole lot better than my five years of psychobabble.

The positive words and actions of other people, as well as our own positive self-talk, are what build our dams. On the other hand, the negative words and actions of other people, as well as our own negative self-talk, are what fill our pools of cess. Throughout our lives, words are the building blocks that program us for better and for worse. Therefore, words are powerful tools to help us debug those programs that promote our cess or weaken our dams. The right words, at the right time, spoken by others or us, can undeniably move our minds into more positive directions. Isn't that precisely why we read books like this one?

Initially, most family and friends' self-talk in Cancerville is not the same as what they say to their loved ones. The voice they use with their loved one is usually positive and hopeful. Yet their inner voice is often one of fear and pessimism, full of sentences that start with "OMG…!" or "What if…?" This is neither healthy nor appropriate. The last thing you need to do is weaken your dam and stir your cesspool into further agitation.

For centuries, many philosophers, spiritual leaders, and mental health professionals, as well as everyday people, have come to realize the value of positive thinking and positive self-talk. As far back as 300 BC, Epicurus encouraged positive thinking as a vehicle toward greater happiness. More recently, in 1952, Norman Vincent Peale published his popular book, *The Power of Positive Thinking*,[12] which has sold millions of copies. The popularity of Peale's book and the many others with similar themes demonstrates the appeal of and need for learning how to be positive. Positive self-talk helps us to accomplish that goal.

There have been naysayers as well. They have preached a more negative and pessimistic set of beliefs. They can be summed up by the sad statement, "Life sucks and then you die." Sometimes, that is most unfortunately true. Then again, the more one feels that way, the more likely these self-fulfilling prophecies will come true, over and over again.

As is my nature, I am trying to strike a balance between your being overly optimistic or overly pessimistic. Realism deals with what is, and optimism deals with what can hopefully be. It accepts, at times with pain-filled disappointment, that into each life some rain will fall. It takes the good with the not-so-good and creates a more comfortable blend of how to look at the world. I hope you can relate and embrace this philosophy too. It can help buffer all the twists and turns in the road, in both life and Cancerville.

The Power of Our Thoughts

Albert Ellis, Ph.D., was an important contributor to the field of psychology and helped change our understanding of human emotion. He was a prolific writer who published many books including the popular *A Guide to Rational Living.*[13] Dr. Ellis founded the Rational Emotive Therapy (RET) school of thought in the 1950s and spent the rest of his career studying, writing, and lecturing about his beliefs, as well as helping many people as a therapist. His later works speak of Rational Emotive Behavioral Therapy (REBT). Ellis teaches us (I was fortunate to have attended one of his lectures while in college) that it is not our emotions that influence our thoughts, as other psychologists believe, but the other way around. He, along with others who founded the Cognitive-Behavioral movement, realized that our thoughts directly and powerfully influence our feelings. To me, our thoughts and our self-talk are one and the same.

Dr. Seligman, whom I referenced in Chapter 4, points out that the question of whether we should talk to ourselves optimistically or not depends upon the cost of being wrong. This directly translates, in my mind, to the realistic part of realistic optimism. The example he uses considers being optimistic about driving home after drinking too much at a party. The cost for that unrealistic optimism can be injury or death to self or others, or a serious DUI. Obviously, that is much too high a cost and risk. That person needs to be realistically pessimistic and call a cab or phone a friend.

What is the cost of optimistic self-talk and hopeful anticipations in Cancerville? Being optimistic in Cancerville costs nothing unless it is entirely unrealistic, as was my cousin Marilyn's case. If optimism is appropriate, it will make your journey and your loved one's a little easier. It is also possible that optimism may even tip the scales toward your loved one's greater comfort, peace of mind, and survival. On the other hand, the cost of pessimistic self-talk is very high in every possible way.

Dr. Ellis developed a simple ABC model to help his clients understand how their negative beliefs and self-talk created problems for themselves. A is for the adverse activating events that people encounter in life. As we know, Cancerville qualifies as an adversity generator of grand proportion. B is for the beliefs the adversity generates, sometimes automatically. These lead to C, the emotional consequences that arise from the beliefs, which greatly influence our feelings, behaviors, and choices. Ellis taught his clients to replace their negative beliefs with more positive and optimistic ones. He and his colleagues were alert for those negative beliefs that occurred automatically in response to adversity.

Let's take a look at the ABCs of Cancerville:

The pessimist says...

A: My loved one has cancer.
B: My loved one will not survive.
C: I feel depressed, terrified, anxious, and overwhelmed. I can't deal with this.

The optimist says ...

A: My loved one has cancer.
B: Many people survive these days.
C: Although I am not happy we are here, I am hopeful we will get through it together. I will do all I can to be helpful and supportive.

Even if your mind initially goes the way of the first ABCs, you can learn to work toward bringing it closer to the second, more optimistic view. The tools in Chapter 16, "Cognitive Tools for Taking Charge of Your Mind," will help you to accomplish that.

The Positive Influence of Positive Self-Talk

Research consistently shows that if people speak to themselves in a positive way, more successful results usually occur. For example, when people anticipate positive outcomes and speak reassuringly to themselves before surgery, a big test, giving an important speech, or the like, the results in all cases are measurably better.

Conversely, for those who speak to themselves with anxious and worrisome anticipations, the outcomes are not nearly as successful. The positive news is that Dr. Seligman and his colleagues all over the world found that people whose self-talk and beliefs are negative can be taught optimism and more positive ways of encouraging themselves forward. Seligman's latest book about positive psychology, *Flourish,*[14] as well as his other books, can help you strengthen your optimism and positive self-talk.

To put their extensive findings in simple terms, people can learn to believe that there isn't a black cloud following them around. The more they can see their situation as random, temporary, and resolvable, and the more they can talk to themselves with reassuring and positive words, the more optimistic they can be about their future.

In your situation in Cancerville, if it is appropriate, it is important to view your loved one's illness as temporary, treatable, and due to random external forces that, unfortunately, just happen to some people. This takes you right back to the self-talk mantras I encouraged previously—"Cancer can be cured. Let's just move forward!" This helps you to see it as conquerable and manageable. This healthier, more optimistic, and positive self-talk helps contain your emotional cess, while your loved one's treatments are working to contain his or her cancer cells.

In *Learned Optimism*, Dr. Seligman tells a story of a young boy with cancer who rapidly went from hopeful to hopeless and sadly died within a day. He says, "Such stories are told the world over, frequently enough to inspire the belief that hope is by itself life-sustaining and hopelessness life-destroying." So it's not just that positive self-talk can be helpful and possibly even healing, but that negative self-talk has a profound, unwanted effect that we all would do well to avoid.

A personal example comes to mind. My cousin Alan died in Cancerville from chemo complications because the technology was so limited in the 1970's. He was in his early thirties and left behind a wife and young daughter. My Aunt Nettie, Alan's mother, fell into a deep depression. Every time I saw her over the next few years, she looked as somber and sad as she had the day of his funeral. Within that time, she developed cancer and died shortly thereafter. It was as if she willed herself to be reunited with her son. There was no doubt in my mind that her chronically depressed state, negative self-talk, and overall misery over the loss of her son lowered her immune system and allowed that to happen.

Fortunately, there are more positive stories shared by Dr. Seligman as well. One involved a research project with people dealing with colon cancer and melanoma. In addition to their regular chemotherapy and radiation treatments, patients received weekly cognitive therapy. They were taught to deal with change, recognize and dispute (remember this word for Chapter 16) automatic pessimistic thoughts, and use distraction techniques. This was supplemented with relaxation training. The goal was to see whether or not these efforts could raise patients' immune systems to help fight off their cancer cells.

These forty people were matched with a control group dealing with the same type of cancers, but who received no cognitive therapy or relaxation. The results were quite impressive. For those who received the additional therapy, their natural killer cell count (the good army) was sharply increased. For those who did not receive the therapy, there was no increase in that cell activity.

Additional research in Cancerville using larger samples also supports the idea that positive beliefs and feelings are beneficial. It makes sense, really, when you consider that the mind and body are directly connected in so many ways. As Susan said, "All of our cells communicate with each other all of the time. That is how the body and mind work together to form a whole and integrated person."

Self-Talk in Cancerville

Please understand that I am not encouraging you to embrace positive self-talk because, if you pass it on to your loved one, it will directly influence his or her outcome; it may or may not have that potential influence. I am, however, encouraging you in that direction because it can help make your time in Cancerville a little easier and much less stressful; it will help you cope better. It will also give you increased energy, greater emotional strength, more patience, a stronger focus, and a brighter outlook.

I do not mean to be unrealistic about this most challenging goal of keeping one's spirits up in Cancerville. Just yesterday, I was talking to Susan, who reminded me again just how difficult it is to stay upbeat and optimistic there. She was coming undone and said:

> My CA-125 numbers are not low enough and I struggle with pain; I'm a mess for more than a week after chemo. Why am I even bothering? I'm going to die from this. I'm tired and I just don't feel good. Look how positive Gilda was, and it didn't do her any f'in' good!

It was hard to argue with Susan's misery and negativity, but I chose to do just that, while understanding and being sensitive to her angst. I spoke to her about adding to her torment by allowing these thoughts to sneak past her dam and generate even more emotional turbulence. I encouraged her to assume that she will be one of the lucky survivors and to see her aches, pain, and hair loss post-chemo as hurting the enemy cells as well. She seemed to embrace that idea.

After our meeting, I had a break and went to Morakami Japanese Gardens, not far from my Boca Raton, Florida office. It is a lush place filled with foliage, relaxing images, and an interesting history. I sat on a bench with a beautiful view of a calming green landscape and pondered our meeting. As a therapist, I often have important responsibilities in areas that are far from clear. I take this responsibility very seriously. I consciously refuse to play God or overstep my boundaries. Just as my degree did not come with a vaccine, neither did it come with a crystal ball.

I asked myself if I was being fair and appropriate to encourage Susan with such a positive agenda under circumstances that were less than positive. Was I promoting unrealistic, naïve, and distorted beliefs? Was I giving her false hope and setting her up for disappointment? I weighed the issues back and forth in my mind like a college debater in a tournament. Yet I ultimately concluded that the preponderance of evidence was on the side of "balls to the walls" positivity in Cancerville, especially for this strong woman.

Part of Susan's difficulty, which applies to family and friends as well, is that at certain times Cancerville can wear down even the strongest of us, both physically and emotionally. This is why we tumble and have to work hard to get back up on that horse named "Hope." When we are drained, distraught, and distracted, working hard is not all that easy, but I believe you can do it. Simply stated, the more positive self-talk you can muster, the less worn you will be, and the more you will be able to focus on what needs to be done.

I would like you to recall times in your life when you rose to a challenge. In one way or another, you have been doing that since you were old enough to walk and talk, perhaps even before. Walking and talking were no easy feats to accomplish back then. Look how far you have come since those early challenges and how many others you have taken on and overcome since then.

I am here reminded of that special little train who willed himself up that high hill by saying, "I think I can, I think I can," as he huffed and puffed himself all the way to the top. Like that little engine, your positive thoughts and self-talk will provide the fuel for you to have the energy to manage Cancerville as well as you can.

Please understand that assuming and believing that your loved one will be a survivor helps make your journey just a little easier. Antje, a cancer survivor for twenty-plus years says, "Be strong in Cancerville, and if it all starts to get to you be even stronger!"

"Yeah, But..."—A Contrarian Point of View

All of these reasonable and rational words aside, I fully understand that it is not always easy to influence a racing mind gone wild over cells gone wild. I get it—I really do. The dips into more negative thoughts and feelings will occur—especially when your loved one isn't feeling particularly well, is tired and lethargic, is on heavy pain meds or steroids, or is experiencing a physical setback of some kind. All of these whack away and weaken your and your loved one's dams. They also cause much worry, which agitates cesspools. Such shifts create a river of negativity. All you can do during these times is pick yourself up, dust off the cess, and refocus on being positive. Rather than seeing your reaction as failing Penzer's Optimism 101 course, see it instead as par for the Cancerville course.

Despite my strong words encouraging you to remain positive, I can almost hear some of you thinking less than positive thoughts such as the following:

> Okay, Bill. You want me to be positive in a place you have characterized as hell, a torture chamber, and a war zone. Need I say more? Okay, I will continue my rant. My loved one's life is in danger, and I am terrified. As you have said, Cancerville operates in slow motion as my mind races along at one hundred and fifty miles per hour, wondering how we got here and how/if we will ever get out. Really, Bill, you expect me to be positive? I think I'd rather be dead myself right now. How's that for positivism? I know you mean well, but buddy, you're way off base!

I do understand those feelings. You have every right to feel the way you do. As your friend, companion, and supporter in Cancerville, I would like to encourage you to move beyond that kind of negative thinking for the sake of your sanity. Yes, have those negative thoughts if they come along (I know I did), but then allow them to pass through your mind and evaporate.

Try to see Cancerville through the more positive self-talk filters of hopefulness, not because I said so, but because that positive attitude may just help you to feel a little better. Yes, my wife and I both selfishly wished we were dead in the early times of our Cancerville arrival. "Selfishly" is definitely the key word in that sentence. As you will come to see, our lives have improved since those dark days. It is certainly possible, and I would like you to optimistically and positively believe that your and your loved one's lives will too.

More Evidence for Hopefulness

Susan not only lent me the *Cure* magazine article referenced in the previous chapter, but also another gem from *Forbes* magazine, March 2, 2009. I chuckled out loud when I read the headline printed boldly on the cover— "Sharon... was 24 and dying from cancer. Then her tumors melted away. What science is learning from... *Miracle Survivors*." The article describes several people with very serious forms of cancer who were told to prepare for their lives to conclude within a few months.

In each case, they experienced an unexpected and complete recovery. Their cancer had totally disappeared. Some were spontaneous remissions, while others were from experimental medications. In all instances, something empowered these patients' immune systems to take charge, tame, and eventually eliminate those ugly cells. Positive self-talk combined with new treatments and a little luck may just have the potential to turn immune systems into superheroes.

The reason for my chuckle was that the article validated the conclusion I had reached sitting on the sunny bench earlier that day in the gardens, while I struggled with how best to help Susan and others in Cancerville. If people sitting on a very precarious perch in Cancerville can make a comeback to solid ground, then we can't pessimistically count almost anyone out.

Accordingly, if a Cancerville doctor told me that I only had a few months to live, my most appropriate and optimistic response would be, "Maybe, maybe not! I'll wait and see what happens." Since miracles and Hail Mary passes only occur on occasion, I would hope and pray for one, while I realistically put my affairs in order and bid my farewells.

In Sum

I fully understand that people in Cancerville will struggle with staying in the positive zone. Like I did, you will have periods of positivism followed by times of worry, upset, and yes, pessimism, hopelessness, and negativity. I encourage you to increase the former and reduce the latter whenever possible. No one expects you or your loved one to always be in good spirits. My hope is to help you talk to yourself in more positive ways more of the time.

I want you to try everyday to do everything you can to look past the negativity of this place and believe it is only temporary, conquerable, and life-saving. You need to try your best to see your loved one as a survivor. It is important to do that for your physical and emotional well-being, as well as for your loved one.

The more you can embrace realistic optimism and its helpful sidekick, positive self-talk, the less difficult and demanding your time in Cancerville will be and the more you will be able to be there for your loved one in every way possible.

Let's move on to help you use more positive self-talk to calm your fears and anxieties. Cancerville is, undeniably, a scary place, but that doesn't automatically mean you have to be panicked there.

CHAPTER 12

I will strengthen my voice of reassurance.

Calming Your Fears and Anxieties

Cancer is the proverbial "monster" hiding quietly in the back of the closet until it comes out and enters your life. At that moment, it becomes an anxiety-provoking force and a source of much tension and terror. It overwhelms you because it has your loved one in its grip.

I want to help you get a grip and assume that with your loved one's medical team leading the way, Cancerville's hold will greatly lessen over time. The power of positive self-talk, which we just discussed, is very helpful in calming your anxieties, as it guides you toward more optimistic beliefs. Remember that little engine and jump on board as we slowly climb up the steep hills of Cancerville saying: "I know I can, I know I can!" I choose to believe that you can.

When Two Scary Places Collide

As I have openly shared with you, I entered Cancerville in a highly charged emotional state. Just return briefly to the Introduction to get back in touch with my overwhelming angst. Frankly, I doubt you want to read that again. I certainly don't; both Ronnie and I cringed whenever it was time to edit that part of the book. For me, Cancerville started as a rough ride, which makes the, introduction a rough read. Upon arrival into Cancerville I was exploding emotionally, like a grenade. Of course, Ronnie won't let me put that word in, once again, before "exploding," but I do believe that it belongs. Go ahead and insert it into the text on your own. You don't have to listen to Ronnie—but I do.

In Chapter 9, "How Minds Work," I also shared how and why, once again, my dam collapsed and my cesspool flooded over upon entering Cancerville. This was because of how I had been programmed from early on and the many losses I had experienced over the intervening years. Anxiety was dripping all over my mind and body and stripping me of much needed energy. I crashed into the wall surrounding Cancerville and burst into flames like an out of control racecar at the Indy 500. Like the affirmation says, I worked hard to find my voice of reassurance. In this chapter I am trying hard to encourage and help you find yours.

Like Anxietyville, Cancerville can be its own unique chamber of agitating inner torment. In Cancerville, your worries and concerns are typically based in reality. They are not ridiculous, distorted, or exaggerated, as they are in Anxietyville. Cancerville is frightening for good reason. Your challenge, however, is to keep your fears from becoming overwhelming. When that happens, your mind races and your mood rapidly declines. You can't engage comfortably in the most basic functions such as eating, sleeping, talking clearly, planning, or managing all the demands of Cancerville. If that happens, you may need some added professional help, a support group, or meds, but let's try to prevent such an overload from shutting down your emotional circuit breakers. You just can't afford to have a blackout, or even a brownout.

The way I converted from terrified to tolerant in Cancerville was by following just about all of the suggestions you will find in this book. I journaled every night, did relaxation exercises, reined in my rage, stopped the pity party, built up my voice of positivism and reassurance, and took charge of my emotional system. I also kept my sense of humor and distracted myself in helpful and healthy ways. I came to own the land in the same way I want you to strive to do. Slowly, but surely, I became "DAM STRONG!" and I want you to feel that way too.

Your goal in Cancerville is to try to manage your stresses and fears and to not get caught up in any serious or disruptive levels of anxiety, such as panic attacks and the like. The former are difficult enough to cope and deal with on a daily basis; the latter can be crippling.

Taking Care of You—Too

Avoiding high levels of anxiety requires taking better care of you. I know you are focused on taking care of and helping your loved one, but your well-being is an important part of the equation. I have observed that when people let themselves go, their anxieties rise as their dam falls and fails to contain their cess. Surely, I was the poster boy in that department; I speak from experience! I am not bragging but just admitting that, at times, my dam was sagging and I was gagging on a mouthful of angst. I am hopeful that won't happen to you. However, if it does, I am optimistic you will be able to use my words and suggestions to strengthen your dam quickly—just as I did.

Try to take better care of you in the simplest of ways. Make sure to eat something on a regular basis, even if it is light. Try to get adequate sleep to recharge your "dam" batteries. Seek out dam supports such as those that will be described in Part IV or any others that can help you to disengage or be distracted from Cancerville whenever you can. Answer your anxieties with a voice that reassures you of positive, day-at-a-time steps forward. By all means, bypass the "bars" in cancer centers or outside them and any other forms of glop. Those may temporarily reduce your anxiety, but they will then take it up a notch or three. I know this all sounds easier said than done, but try your best to get it done. Healthfully supporting yourself will help you better support your loved one.

Though it is not always possible, try to avoid people, places, and things that agitate your cess. That said, I fully understand that some of the people in Cancerville, the place itself, and the things that happen there are all major agitators. This is all the more reason to escape from time to time, in any healthy way that you can, and to draw upon the tools and supports that I will discuss in Part IV.

In addition, be aware of the anxiety generated when we feel "stuck" in any way. In Cancerville, the likelihood is you will feel very stuck and trapped in a place you don't want to be. Those feelings make sense, really. Reducing your feelings of being stuck is part of taking care of yourself. It will be calming and salving for you to think about your stressful time there as being temporary. In addition, picturing more pleasant and positive scenes beyond Cancerville will enable you to visualize you and your loved one getting back to more comfortable times. The more you can see the proverbial "light at the end of the tunnel," the less you will feel stuck and trapped inside the tunnel.

Making Fear Work for You

As anyone who has experienced high levels of anxiety can attest, those uncomfortable and overwhelming feelings consume a great deal of energy and block a person from operating at full capacity. The unknown, and all that goes with it, typically pushes anxieties to all-time levels of intensity. Because Cancerville is most definitely unknown central, you may experience some of the highest levels of anxiety you have ever encountered. At the very time you need all the energy, focus, and coping you can muster, anxiety becomes a force with which you need to reckon.

Trying to reassure yourself becomes an undeniable challenge, but one that you can achieve. Dig deep inside by reminding yourself of other times in your life that your skeptical, negative voice of doubt tried to take charge. Realize that it was not an accurate voice then and isn't necessarily now. You can override it with a more realistically optimistic and reassuring voice at this time.

During times in the past when your anxiety took over, you probably compensated by increasing your effort. You studied, worked, and tried harder to do your best to prevent your anxious and negative anticipations from influencing the results. In all likelihood, most of the time you achieved your goal.

Though you don't have as much control in Cancerville, your fear can serve a similar purpose. It will motivate you to be present, focused, and on top of everything you can be for your loved one. Your fear will also convert to action, which, as we have already discovered, is your trump card to override difficult emotional times. When in doubt, do something helpful. Or just do something, and hope it will be helpful. Remember "Pinky" power. Had I known then what I know now, I would have bought a "Pinky" for Ronnie and one for me as well.

Rob's fear motivated him to move his son to Sloan-Kettering. Remember that his worries also motivated him to contact doctors at other major cancer centers to make sure that they agreed with the treatment protocol being used. His terror motivated him to do all of those things I told you about in Chapter 2. Fear pushes us to adapt, take charge, and take on Cancerville with all of our might. It is those very fearful feelings that improve our slingshot aim. Our hands may sweat and shake at times, but our aim is right on target.

Similarly, Susan's initial fears had her welcoming the surgery that would get those cells out of her ASAP. Subsequent fears about the chemo protocols not working sent her to different cancer centers to obtain additional feedback regarding trials that could help fight off her aggressive cells.

A dentist in Israel by profession, Dani's fear transformed him into a very knowledgeable scientist who studied multiple issues about his multiple myeloma. He is the poster person for the doctor/patient partnership as he has played a very active role in his treatment program. He far outlived his doctor's predictions. Many have shared with me that their anxieties gave them the strength and courage to endure major and painful surgery, disruptive chemotherapy, and whatever else was required in their search for the cure.

I never asked Jodi, but my guess is her fears brought out the sure-footed parts that allowed her to dance the most demanding "routine" of her life with energy and grace. My fears led me to challenge my initial meltdown every step of the way and work hard to override my earlier cesspool programming. Ronnie's fears motivated her to be present at every doctor meeting, armed with her list of questions. Fears and anxieties can paralyze us if we allow them to, or they can energize us to rise to new heights. Each of us has many choices in how we overcome our fears and "power up" our voice of reassurance.

The previous two chapters, on optimism and positivism, can be drawn upon as counterforces to your anxieties. Whenever possible, use them as vaccines to insulate, inoculate, and immunize yourself so all that worry can be kept, if not completely in check, at least in balance. Talk to yourself as you would reassuringly talk to and encourage a friend in a similar position. Reassure yourself, realistically, that all will likely be well.

For those whose voice of reassurance has never been that strong, know that it can be strengthened just as optimism can be learned. I believe Dr. Seligman would agree that being able to be self-reassuring is an important part of becoming more optimistic. Start by talking positively to yourself, even if you don't believe all that you are saying. Keep talking that way, repeating the self-reassuring, positive self-talk mantras. Sooner than later, you will become more of a believer in the power and credibility of your own words.

Getting to Calmer Space

I know personally that it is definitely possible to start out in the sky is falling—Chicken Little—position and move slowly, but surely, toward soaring like an eagle. We are very adaptive, especially as we rise to take on Cancerville. Even if you catch yourself moving in a less than positive or reassuring direction, you can reverse course. You can gently bring yourself back to more neutral and reassuring thoughts and feelings.

Try to consistently flood your mind with positives. Think about the credentials of your medical team and their earnest efforts and determined, dedicated devotion to your cause. Focus on the research teams discovering new treatments and better ways to deliver them; think about the miracle cures and spontaneous remissions. Today I read about a man in Germany who was diagnosed three years ago with leukemia and HIV. The doctors mixed multiple treatments together, and he is now free of both diseases. He is the first person to be cured of HIV. Remind yourself that new technology is continuously entering Cancerville to shore up and expand its present artillery.

Think about all of the different heavies that you never, ever think about the way you have been thinking, worrying, and obsessing about Cancerville. Coincidentally, a man who looked to be in his forties just passed by where I am sitting and writing the above words. He could barely walk as he, not so easily, dragged three hundred and fifty or more pounds along. He didn't appear to be worried and anxious that he might drop in his slow tracks at any moment. Nor does he appear to be depressed to the point of missing a meal. The woman walking with him did not seem terrified or down about what appeared to be his serious risk factors either.

Some of us face far more real and present dangers to our lives every day than Cancerville poses and don't give them serious thought or concern. Even Dr. Oz admitted to dragging his tush to avoid getting his colonoscopies in a timely or protective basis. I admire his effort to get us off our butts by being so forthright.

Gaining Strength from Your Loved One

Another source of reassurance can come from the strength of your loved one. Estelle, Dani's wife, said, "Our strengths played off each other. He never complained, was easygoing, proactive, and always hopeful. He gave me strength and courage and we also prayed a lot."

Shelly, my colleague for many years, told me that her husband, Mike, was diagnosed right after they were married. She said, "He was the most positive, optimistic person I knew and always believed the treatment would work. That was contagious for me and helped me through the many ordeals we experienced. He helped me to become a stronger, and more positive cheerleader for him.

Over and over again, I have observed people with cancer becoming even stronger than they were before. Just about all the people I've known who were diagnosed with cancer have met Cancerville squarely and head-on. Although Jodi may have cried those understandable elephant tears while walking to the operating room, overall she demonstrated a degree of strength in Cancerville that raised the bar for facing and owning its land. My daughter stared it down better than I could have!

Jodi sucked it up, rarely complained, and moved steadily forward like the beautiful and spirited dancer she has always been. She followed the chorus line of Cancerville gracefully, just as she has done in all areas of her life. Rob's twin sons, Jake and Chase, showed this same strength and courage as well. Most of the time they responded like adults, despite being only eight-and-a-half years old. The same is true of Susan, Phil, Antje, Carol, Howie, Eileen, Terry, Marcy, Dani, Shelley, Mike, and all of the other people going through Cancerville that I've had the privilege of knowing. People with cancer show their physical and emotional muscle over and over again in a very courageous fashion.

In an unexpected way, your loved one's strengths will fuel your own. This is true even if your loved one is a little boy or girl. Hopefully, you will admire and strive to emulate your loved one's courage and determination as he or she bravely copes with and tolerates the stresses of Cancerville and the demands of treatment.

In Sum

Please work hard in all ways to prevent Cancerville from weighing you down with high levels of anxiety. I fully understand that striving to steer your mind out of fearful, anxiety-provoking space is not easy. Remember, I am the poster man for panic during my Anxietyville days, as well as anxiety during my early Cancerville time.

I remember how difficult it was to counterpunch and contain my cesspool that was filled with a lifetime of anxious anticipations and pessimistic feelings—but I did. You can, too, by scoring some Rocky-esque knockout punches to that old fearful cess, as well as to those issues in Cancerville that are frightening you in the present. I am simply encouraging you to try your hardest to push your mind away from your fears, and align much more with your loved one's strength and his or her doctor's might.

Now, let's take a look at yet another potentially destructive emotion that can also drain much needed energies. Let's help you get quickly past any guilt you may be feeling. It is a common reaction but one that is uncalled for and undeserved in Cancerville. Your loved one's cancer is not your fault. Period!

CHAPTER 13

It is not my fault that my loved one has cancer.

Getting Past Your Guilt

Though you are extremely upset that your loved one is in Cancerville, I hope you realize that it is not your fault in any way. Despite my emotional upheaval, that was my feeling throughout. I never knowingly did anything to hurt any of my children. I doubt you ever did either. You certainly don't need or deserve any guilt added to your already agitated cesspool. If you are free of any guilt and clear on that issue, you can skip this chapter completely. If, on the other hand, you are feeling any guilt at all, please continue reading, as I want to help you let it go.

It is easy to feel guilty in Cancerville, especially if you are the parent of the patient. Parents and others close to the patient feel they should have protected him or her. As I previously said, watch out for "should" statements. They are typically exaggerated and inaccurate.

Within seconds of hearing the diagnosis, you can feel as though it is your fault. "If only I did..." or "If only I didn't..." thoughts can rapidly race through your mind. Please try not to do that to yourself. Your feelings of guilt, false as they might be, will drain you of energy. They will torture and torment you and will rob you of the positive power you need in Cancerville. Guilt is undeniably a form of emotional kryptonite that is inappropriate. The sooner you can move away from it, the better you will feel and the more you can do to be helpful.

A Primer on Guilt's Origins and Purpose

People are taught guilt from the time that they are very young. Listen to yourself as a parent or listen to other parents in public places. "How could you?" "You are a bad boy/girl." "I am ashamed of you." "Because you did that we aren't going to...." "Look how nicely your sister is behaving." "What's wrong with you?"

When I hear those kinds of statements in public, I often wonder what these moms or dads say in private. In moderate doses, gentler feedback can help build a conscience that serves as a moral compass to guide us through life. They help us choose pride bank deposits instead of shame and blame ones. In excess, however, overdoing guilt causes us to overdose and feel too much is all our fault, even when we don't deserve to feel that way. As I have often said, the proverbial guilt-inducing "Jewish Mother" comes in all religions. Recently, the idea of "tiger moms" seems to have turned *Portnoy's Complaint* into an internationally relevant issue.

As my buddy Siggie taught us, we all have an id (wild child), ego (adult manager), and superego. The latter is our conscience and the seat and center of our guilt-strings. The superego is created by society as taught by our parents, teachers, and all the other annoying people who tried to show us right from wrong. These are the well-meaning people whose sentences started with "Don't," "How dare you?" and "I can't believe you ate the whole thing."

The important issue to understand from all of this is that, in moderation, guilt serves us well and keeps us out of harm's way. It puts an emergency brake on our "child" parts that would like to run glopfully wild. But it serves no purpose when unreasonable and undeserved self-blame makes us feel badly. Try to avoid those self-defeating, self-deflating feelings generally, and particularly in Cancerville.

Different people feel different degrees of guilt. Some experience excessive guilt and feel most negative things are their fault. Others have a "guilt deficiency disorder" and would do well to borrow some from the first group. Fortunately, there are many people who have appropriate levels of guilt. This enables them to manage their lives appropriately and color within the lines. They follow the "rules," do the right thing, and avoid putting themselves in harm's way. That is the way it is supposed to be in order to fill pride banks.

Some people, like those in the first group mentioned above, are masters at self-defeatingly twisting and turning life's problems into a guilt attack that reeks of "shouda," "coulda," and "woulda" toxins. If you find yourself in this group, try to remember, first and foremost, that you could not have prevented your loved one from getting sick. Second, if you could have, you would have! In fact, you would have done anything and everything to prevent your loved one from entering Cancerville. And now you will do anything and everything you can to help your loved one get through Cancerville.

Let these simple statements salve your guilt. Realistically, I understand that simple statements do not immediately resolve complex emotional issues, but I put them here, optimistically, for you to consider. You can reread them over and over until they help you finally let go of your Cancerville-related guilt.

No One Cause and No One Knows the Cause

Cancer is a product of random forces all happening together in a perfect-storm way. Think dominoes collapsing upon one another here. Think cancer cells sitting quietly dormant for many years or even decades and then, all of a sudden, bursting loose. Think cells gone wild in a flash. There are many variations of Cancerville's graceless repertoire.

Even when there are genetic linkages, they are complicated, confusing, and definitely beyond your control or responsibility. Whether you heated things in plastic, fed your loved one char-grilled burgers, or did something else for which you now feel guilty, please don't blame yourself. Carcinogens exist everywhere, and research findings have been inconsistent. Even the research that clearly links smoking to cancer does not explain why some pack-or-more-a-day smokers can live till eighty something and why both Dana Reeves and my cousin Marilyn got lung cancer even though they never smoked. Go figure!

There is yet another related issue that showers guilt on family members like a 3 p.m. Florida rainstorm in July. It is similar to what people often feel after a disaster when others did not survive but they did. It occurs when you wish that you, not your loved one, had cancer. This scenario is particularly prevalent among parents who would step in front of the Cancerville bullet in a heart-filled beat. Older grandparents and even friends can experience similar guilt-based feelings. My mother was ninety-five and was doing well when Jodi was diagnosed, and it seemed so ridiculously unfair and inequitable to me. Please don't get me wrong; I loved my mother, but "this cannot be my daughter's turn!"

Part of just about every parent's unwritten "protective policy" is to allow no evil to affect his or her child, no matter the child's age. Should something happen to our child, we wish it happened to us. Unfortunately, it doesn't work that way, as tragedy and trauma are not transferable. In this realm we have no control. Read that last sentence over again and embrace it to stop your guilt in its tracks. You had no control or influence over your loved one developing cancer. That is a fact.

Despite all of my appeals directed to the jury of your mind, I understand that some are prone to guilt automatically and irreversibly. Despite her being a loyal and committed daughter, person, partner, and parent, Ronnie suffered totally undeserved guilt as we traveled through Cancerville. The details are not important. She was raised by parents who imposed a harsh conscience.

As a result of her upbringing, Ronnie's cesspool quickly takes her to guilt generally, and especially when it comes to those she loves. Her devotion to me and to our children and grandchildren, as you may have already sensed, is extremely strong. You better believe that she would have been first in line if Jodi's cancer cells were transferable. Even though I am not a guilt-ridden person, I would have jumped in front of her if it were possible to spare our daughter from going through Cancerville. I'm quite sure that many reading this book feel the same way.

My words only partially helped Ronnie let go of her feelings of guilt. I imagine she has carried those inappropriate feelings forward, even as we have done our best to distance ourselves from Cancerville. Try your best to use my words to help you leave your guilt behind. In this regard, I hope you can do even better than Ronnie.

In Sum

It is not your fault that your loved one developed cancer, but you can help your loved one now. This is no time for guilt of any kind. This is the time to confront and take charge of a very painful reality that has grabbed hold of your loved one.

Cancer is a random event that can choose the healthiest and fittest among us. It makes no sense really, but that is the case for so many difficult experiences that we can encounter. It takes us right back to the unfairness of life. But given those unavoidable inequities, try your best not to be unfair to yourself.

Let's move on to tackle yet another emotional challenge. Your anger will likely flow in Cancerville at different times or all of the time; you might just need to rein it in.

CHAPTER 14

I will not allow anger to drain me.

Reining in Your Rage

Everyone experiences angry feelings from time to time. Anger is a universal emotion. How we choose to express our anger and whether we manage it appropriately is a reflection of our emotional balance. When a person is screaming, cursing, or punching walls, rest assured that cess is bursting through the dam like a spring flash flood in the Midwest.

Just about everyone in Cancerville feels angry. I do not believe you or your loved one can be there without periodically feeling and expressing some of that emotion. Everything about Cancerville arouses primal rage. It is an affront to your sensibilities and sensitivities, as it is contrary to all you have come to believe about fair play, especially as that applies to your loved one. I want to explain why this is so and, as importantly, discuss what you can do to keep your anger at more manageable levels.

The Basis of Anger

Generally, people become angry and/or enraged in reaction to the following experiences:

- abuse
- insults
- inequity
- inconsideration
- irrationality
- disappointment
- hurtful consequences
- the unknown
- loss of control

We all want and expect to be treated fairly and kindly, and we want the same for our loved ones. We feel this is what we deserve. While we may all define "deserve" differently in other circumstances, it is likely that in Cancerville we are in much agreement. Just about no one deserves to be in Cancerville or be faced with all that goes with it.

In one way or another, Cancerville has the potential to create just about every issue on the above list. Those are what will fuel your anger, and those are what fueled mine. Cancer is not supposed to happen to our loved ones, and life is supposed to be fair to them. All is supposed to go smoothly and well, and our loved ones should be able to all live happily ever after.

These strong but distorted beliefs help us feel safe and secure while wrapped in our delusional blankie. That it has nothing to do with reality is beside the point. When Cancerville rips that blankie away, we react with the same fury and protest as people who are being denied their basic human rights and freedom. In fact, Cancerville is not a democratic place. It is an autocratic, demanding, restricting, and, at times, even punishing place. How could we not be enraged by all of that?

The raging, righteous indignation that I felt, not only on July 8, 2005, but also throughout Jodi's treatment, was based upon a powerful but false belief. Its origin is reflected clearly in my "This cannot be my daughter's turn" inner scream of denial and lament. I, like most, held on to the strong but inaccurate belief that bad things happen to other people—not to me, my wife, and certainly not to any of my children or grandchildren. It took a while for me to realize the error of my thinking. Susan raised this same issue but quickly realized it was irrational. She said, "I sit here and ask myself how this happened to me, and then I ask myself why shouldn't this have happened to me? What makes me different from anyone else who gets cancer? Cancer happens to people, and I am a person."

In Chapter 1, I referred to these kinds of distortions as belonging to a form of healthy denial because they allow us all to move freely about the planet. They also allow us to believe that our loved ones will do the same. As I have said, this healthy denial enables us to function in our daily lives. If we sat around and obsessively worried about car crashes, we wouldn't give our children the keys to the family car or even have one. If we sat around worrying about the next Columbine incident, all children would be homeschooled. We would be labeled hypochondriacs if we sat around and worried about cancer or any other serious disease. When our necessary but inaccurate denial is pierced with negative news of any kind, especially a cancer diagnosis, the result is raging disbelief and disapproval.

Anger and Angst in Cancerville

How could you not be angry or at least feel some angst from time to time that you and your loved one have been forced to enter Cancerville? How could you not resent the intrusion of all of Cancerville's worries, stresses, and cess to your already existing load? Moreover, how can you bypass the bitter and enraged feelings that your loved one is being put through harsh treatments and has been placed in harm's way? Who wouldn't be furious that Cancerville is a reality for you and your loved one? For those who like to say everything happens for a reason, I'd like them to explain the reason anyone is forced to enter Cancerville. The only reason I can fathom is the randomness of life and cancer cells. It is like hitting a lousy—a really lousy—lottery.

Beyond your initial upset that you and your loved one are in Cancerville, there are so many possible happenings that will add to your anger and fuel your rage. These include the treatments (some of which may have painful or uncomfortable side effects), waiting to see the doctor, mindboggling bills (independent of whether your loved one, you, or insurance are paying them), medical miscues, insensitive comments by hospital staff that are unwittingly made, inadequate and depressing facilities, chemo that doesn't work the way it is supposed to, and so much more.

The Need to Suppress and Express

Talking about insensitive and/or inappropriate comments, a few months after Jodi's surgery, I asked a receptionist a simple question. In response, she made an insensitive comment, which made no sense relative to my question. I, a quiet man, had some pretty angry thoughts. For the good of the cause, I just retreated into the sea of people in the waiting room. That there were so many people in that room was heart-wrenching enough. Sometimes a held tongue is the better option. Whatever I said would have included words Ronnie would not allow me to use in this book. So one coping strategy is just to not get into it, tempting as that might be.

Many people tend to store anger like a squirrel stores nuts. For the squirrel, that behavior gets him through a cold winter. For us, there are times when we need to store and suppress the anger to get us through a potentially cold and hurtful scene. Most if not all of the time, going nuts does more harm than good. Yet it needs to be released in some way, as storing it is unhealthy. That angry cess builds up over time and eventually we implode or explode from its weighty force.

To release the anger I had suppressed toward the receptionist, I journaled like a madman that night because I was a very mad man. It felt good to get it out of my cesspool in an appropriate rant. This helped me let go of it and just move forward! It is important for you to know that there are many avenues to release and vent, only one of which is direct confrontation.

Walking around with a nuclear chip on your shoulder is not conducive to being calm and comfortable. On the contrary, all that chip does is weigh you down and cover your day-to-day life with toxic waste. Those who do store rage regularly often end up with ulcers, high blood pressure, heart attacks, or other physical problems.

In addition to all of the above, anger and rage can too easily lead and feed into depression. Though we no longer glibly talk about depression being anger turned inward, anger is still a turbulent force with which to reckon. When that anger has no place to go, it can also turn against us; it fuels our fury and can become an excuse to do glop. All of our angst can seek out a variety of self-destructive "vents" like a moth heading for a flame. In a counterproductive way, all this does is make everything more difficult and fill us with even more self-directed rage, as well as shame and blame feelings. It is important that we be alert and watch out for vicious cycles of any kind. In life and especially in Cancerville, we need positive cycles.

The Importance of Venting Cess

As you already know, your cesspool wasn't exactly empty before you entered Cancerville. In fact, the likelihood is that it was pretty full, if not overflowing. Adding Cancerville angst to all of that existing cess is likely to send a very strong tidal wave toward your dam, like a tsunami heading right for a slumbering village. It is important, if not imperative, that your dam stands tall during your time in Cancerville, despite the tumult going on inside you. The key to maintaining balance between your cesspool and your dam is to vent your accumulated cess in whatever healthy way is comfortable for you.

Rob raged on his blog about his son's school not allowing him to set up a videoconference so that Jake, at Sloan-Kettering, could have a chat with his chums. He knew the principal would likely see the blog, but he didn't care. But then, in his signature style, Rob took it a step further. He arranged for several of the children to come to his house and did the video chat from there. He first vented his anger and then channeled it into a constructive action that accomplished his original goal. That one-two combination is a healthy way to deal with anger. In many instances, taking action neutralizes your anger by getting something done, rather than your coming undone.

Similarly, when we spoke yesterday, Susan was furious. She was angry at cancer, Cancerville, her pains and fatigue, the chemo that wasn't working, and some important blood test results that were a week late. The latter was pushing her over the edge. She dumped her fury and frustrations onto the floor of my office and left with a renewed sense of taking charge of her situation in an empowered way. Dumping cess in appropriate ways helps us to reduce and better manage our anger.

Talking to a psychiatrist, psychologist, social worker, or mental health counselor is an excellent way to vent angry feelings and receive emotional support at the same time. We will talk more about this in Chapter 17, "Having a Counselor and/or Support Group in Your Corner." In addition to counseling, the following are some other examples of healthy ways to vent frustrations and angry feelings:

Verbal Vents:

- joining a support group
- talking to a close friend/relative

Written Vents:

- blogging
- emailing
- social networking
- journaling
- writing poems, articles, or a book

Artistic Vents:

- painting
- sculpting

Personal Exercise:

- working out
- doing yoga
- punching a bag
- walking, jogging, or running
- jumping rope
- swimming
- hitting golf balls

Group Sports:

- tennis
- racquetball
- basketball

Physical Releases:

- crying or laughing
- ripping newspapers
- punching a pillow
- chopping wood
- using a sauna/steam room to sweat it out
- loudly rooting for your home sports team

Any of the above activities or others that release pent-up feelings and frustrations, which are not violent, inappropriate, or glopful, are worth drawing upon during your journey through Cancerville.

My personal experience and professional observations suggest that the more we vent our angers, resentments, and frustrations in healthy ways, the more we can release them safely. This prevents them from becoming toxic and polluting us in ways that ultimately lead to self-defeating behaviors, which then convert to shame and blame deposits. This also protects your dam from being weakened by the stored-up cess.

In addition, venting keeps you from allowing your angers to spill out onto other people, most of whom are innocent bystanders. In hindsight, what would my going off on a well-meaning but harried receptionist who wasn't paying attention have accomplished? It would have attracted the attention of a room full of unhappy people. I would have been seen as and felt like a jerk!

In Sum

I hope this discussion about managing your anger in Cancerville will help you to rein much of your rage and anger. In addition, there are some excellent books and workbooks on anger management that can be supportive.

It is important for you to find appropriate and comfortable ways to vent and release as much cess as possible. Most of the time, those build-ups create a variety of unhealthy and unhelpful consequences. As you now know, too much cess can cause a mess and much stress.

There is yet another way to vent your anger in a healthy way. Send me an email at bill@cancerville.com; it may help you to release pent-up feelings. I promise I will personally respond, not as a therapist, but as your Cancerville friend and support.

Let's move on to Part IV. This provides some simple and practical tools that you can use to be more successful in achieving the emotional goals I have encouraged.

PART IV

Tools That Help You Tend the Land

CHAPTER 15

I will practice relaxing activities whenever I can.

Relaxing Tools for Natural Healing

I wondered where I would write this chapter to fully capture the essence of my message. I have now found that special place. I am sitting in front of my mini-computer aboard a cruise ship that is sailing through Milford Sound, New Zealand at 7 a.m. It is a pristine and peaceful place where mountains and glaciers produce sparkling waterfalls and exceptionally low-lying clouds, even on this gray and chilly morning. All of my senses are awake despite the early hour. Classical music is playing softly in the background. My world seems at peace in this quiet, mostly deserted place.

The Value of Vitaminds and Mental Floss

Although this is a special and unique place, the message of Milford Sound applies to wherever you might be in the world right now and to however you might be feeling today. This message is simply about influencing how you feel by altering your sensory experience.

If for you Cancerville is a cauldron of burning sensations amid jumbled emotions and a deep sense of dread, then the tools in this chapter offer a calmer, gentler, and more peaceful alternative. They encourage you to take a break from Cancerville for a few minutes each day and experience a taste of Tranquilityville. These tools and activities represent the emotional equivalent of vitamins (vitaminds) and dental floss (mental floss). They will strengthen your dam while clearing away the plaque-like build-up of cess from the walls of your mind. They will help lower your anxieties, reduce your feelings of depression, and limit your negative self-talk, while strengthening your voice of hopefulness and optimism. They offer very small doses of peace of mind at a time when those feelings are not easy to achieve.

Most of us are peculiarly paradoxical in a variety of ways. Though many want to feel in control, we don't always take control when those very opportunities present themselves. Hear ye, hear ye, hear ye! The tools and techniques that I am about to describe offer some simple and powerful ways to better control your body and your mind.

Yet just as with taking our vitamins or flossing our teeth, we can be lazy and self-neglecting in the silliest of ways. Many of the tools I will describe only take a few minutes a day to use. Though such a small investment of time can yield such powerful dividends in terms of soothing, calming, and healing feelings, we often short-change ourselves by avoiding them. In our busifying, dizzifying quest to do and achieve, we can forget to just be and relax—even for just a few minutes.

For those in Cancerville, the typical everyday hustle-bustle is accelerated many times over. There is everything that previously needed to be managed, plus all of the logistical challenges of Cancerville, commingled with enough emotional hurdles to make for an Olympic-sized event. For these reasons, we need to create some powerful and positive sensory experiences. These help us offset the less than lovely images that abound and surround us in Cancerville. That you don't have much time is clear; but that you have ten to twenty minutes a day for a vitamind or two or for mental flossing is equally undeniable. You will note, as well, that some of these tools really require no time at all for you to take advantage of their benefits.

Finally, at a time when the words green and organic have become part of our ideal lifestyle, the following tools fit those natural criteria perfectly. None involve foreign or toxic substances. All are as green as the trees and foliage that grow on the soil-less slopes of the mountains of Milford Sound, still visible as our ship moves on to its next vantage point.

In all of the activities that follow, the goal is to soothe, nurture, and heal the agitation of your mind and body. I am quite sure you are already aware of all of the tools I am encouraging you to try. None are profound, complex, or original. I have not discovered these tools, but I have personally and professionally discovered their multiple benefits. I sincerely hope you will too.

Rather than just list these tools, I want to describe my own experiences with them. I do not expect that all of the tools I use and enjoy will fit your needs. Your goal is not to embrace each and every one; ideally, you will find a few that work for you and will draw upon them as often as you can. You may find one or two that you can enjoy with your loved one, which will increase its power and meaningfulness.

Passive and Peaceful Tools

This section describes relaxing sensory experiences that take no time and require little energy. They simply provide a calming background to your environs.

Music

I very much enjoy listening to soothing music, either of the spa, classical, or smooth jazz type. I play that music in my home whenever I am there and listen to it when I walk alone in the park. I also have it playing in the background in my office as well as in the waiting room, along with a relaxing DVD. I have never understood why many doctor and dental offices have CNN blaring when soothing images and sounds would be more helpful.

Most mornings, I like to start my day listening to a spa-like meditational music CD in the little library just off our bedroom. I listen while thinking about everything and nothing at the same time. Sometimes a thought may hit me, and I reach for a yellow pad; mostly, I just try to be there, quietly present in this awakening moment.

Whatever type of music relaxes you is fine. You may prefer classical, inspirational, show tunes, or the like; you might be someone who relaxes by listening to rock or rap. My concern is not which music works for you, but that you choose to use music to influence your mood and brighten your spirit.

Other Calming Sounds

I also use fountains, both at home and at my office, for similar purposes. The sound of flowing water is universally calming. Even people who don't enjoy swimming often seek out the relaxing influence of the beach in order to hear the sound of the waves breaking at the shoreline. Brookstone and other similar stores sell machines that play a variety of calming sounds including the ocean, raindrops hitting the roof, or a babbling brook. Smart phones have apps for these as well. All these sounds can induce peacefulness and sleep.

In this same category of passive influences are relaxing DVDs. These show calming images, such as aquariums, beaches, sunsets, snowfalls, etc., combined with peaceful music. The only effort they require is hitting the remote. They are very helpful in briefly distracting you from Cancerville and giving your mind a rest.

Aromas

In the same vein, I enjoy candles and light them frequently in my office when the fire officials aren't looking. I admit that I failed inspection once because I had one burning in the waiting room. Please don't tell them I still light one on occasion. There is something very captivating about the little dancing flame and the aromatic scents that have a calming influence on our senses. You can experiment to find out which aromas are helpful for you.

Peaceful Spaces

Finally, sometimes calm and peaceful feelings arise when we place ourselves in a soothing environment. This is presently the case for me as our ship continues its journey through Milford Sound. However, it need not be as exotic, as many opportunities exist closer to home.

I previously mentioned going to Morakami Gardens in Delray Beach, Florida, because this large Japanese garden immediately relaxes me. It is Tranquilityville central! The same is true for my time at the beach in Jupiter, Florida, where I do much of my writing while enjoying the relaxing sights and sounds.

Others report similar pleasant sensations and feelings from a sauna, massage, aquarium visit, concert hall symphony, or spiritual sanctuary. My simple encouragement is for you to take a break from Cancerville from time to time and consciously put yourself in an environment that is relaxing for you. It really doesn't matter what places do that for you as long as you seek out safe and calming spaces whenever possible.

I hope you will try to find some passive and peaceful tools from the above examples or look into others that fit your nature and your needs. There are many vitaminds/mental floss from which you can choose to help you take a brief respite from the stressors of Cancerville.

Active Peaceful Tools

The following tools require more active involvement on your part. The good news is that they are user-friendly and very effective in providing peace of mind. The nice part about these tools is that they are portable and completely within your control.

Muscle Relaxation

Progressive/autogenic muscle relaxation is a very simple and effective tool that I first learned about when I worked at Nova University. A colleague taught me this technique in 1973. I was attached via electrodes to a biofeedback machine that measured and provided audio feedback that showed my level of muscle tension. The relaxation technique simply involves tensing and then relaxing each muscle group. It helps people reduce their bodily tensions very easily. I have even used an abbreviated version of autogenic relaxation, without biofeedback, in large audiences, and just about everyone in the room enjoyed the experience.

The goal of this relaxation tool is to create a very calm and peaceful alpha brain state. Portable, hand-held biofeedback machines, as compared to the larger ones of old, are available these days. However, I have found that relaxation exercises work very well without the biofeedback, as some find the sound distracting.

I used muscle tensing and relaxing to successfully calm my own anxiety back in the 1970s and again in 2005, when I was struggling with our journey through Cancerville. I still use it for myself, as well as with people I am currently helping. It has stood the test of time based on its simplicity and effectiveness. There are a variety of CDs available with these types of exercises. This includes my "Zen and Now" remake of a 1980s relaxation tape that has both autogenic and guided imagery exercises. Both are in my voice. There is also a wonderfully relaxing DVD that I made after a recent visit to Iguassu Falls in South America. Both are available at www.cancerville.com.

Guided Imagery

Guided imagery has also been a favorite of mine as a relaxation/distraction tool. I still use it to "escape" the dentist's chair by transporting myself to a different place and time. I let the dentist do his or her thing while I visit the beach, the countryside, or some other peaceful and pleasant scene in my mind's eye. I hope you have some pleasant, peaceful scenes stored in your mind's DVR to which you can occasionally return.

Other Peaceful Activities

I also encourage people in Cancerville to see beyond the moment and begin to picture brighter, happier, more comfortable scenes in the future. Though it would have been impossible for me to imagine my family's own fairy tale, which I shall soon share, I did try my best to see more comfortable days ahead, instead of the difficult ones I faced during Jodi's treatment time.

In addition, mindfulness, meditation, yoga, Qigong, Tai chi, and self-hypnosis are all active peaceful tools. They can be mesmerizing in inducing powerful feelings of calm and peace of mind. They distract from the everyday stressors and help us to focus on the now. Many websites, books, DVDs, mental health professionals, and classes exist that can guide you through these activities.

If you haven't already, I encourage you to explore these tools to see if one can be helpful for you. I do understand, however, that your stressful, task-oriented days generally, and especially in Cancerville, often allow little to no time for relaxation activities. Even though I know you are very busy, I am pushing you to push yourself, from time to time, to take a short relaxation break from Cancerville.

Despite my encouragements, I admit that I have tried several of these pleasant and relaxing activities, but like many people, have not been able to sustain consistent practice and participation. Here, I run right into the doing wall of productive accomplishments that so easily blocks my path. Often, I don't take the time to seek calmer consciousness. An example is what has happened to me this morning. I awoke at 7 a.m. to see and be mindful of the sights of the sound. I found these views and vistas inspiring and quickly started typing rather than just relaxing. Perhaps the answer is that relaxation comes in many different forms for many different people.

Relaxing Distractions

I believe there are times when what we are doing, even if it isn't a specific relaxation exercise or activity, can also contribute to our being calmer and more relaxed. There is no reason to be judgmental about what facilitates our relaxation. For example, isn't it likely that with its clear focus, creative flow, energizing power, and pride bank deposits, writing this morning was as calming for me as being fully mindful of the beautiful vistas?

This leads to the idea that beyond the relaxation exercises I've described, there may be many other activities that can serve a similar purpose for you. Working, working out, or simply having mindless fun can all contribute to calmer feelings. Perhaps your relaxation comes from watching NASCAR, knitting, playing cards, reading, completing a crossword puzzle, or doing something else that you enjoy. I was surprised to learn that the average age of people who play computer games is thirty-seven. In the same vein, the average American watches two and a half hours of TV on weekdays. As long as it is not glopful, it doesn't matter how you recharge your batteries. What matters, especially in Cancerville, is that you do.

Your mind needs some breaks from the tension and tedium. A part of you needs to help yourself disengage from thinking, reading, or talking about Cancerville. You may even want to put down this book and take a break for a while; I will not take it personally.

Try to see these distractions as nutrients for your mind and your dam. That your loved one is in Cancerville may reduce your appetite, but it need not stop you from eating. Neither does it have to stop you from engaging in some emotionally nourishing distractions. Feeding both your body and your mind are very important. Clearly, the choice of distractions is yours as are the many rewards that come as a relief, such as a calming and rebuilding of worn out nerve endings, a rekindling of your spirit, and a renewal of your soul.

A Passive and Essential Inactivity

We tend to take a good night's sleep for granted until we have trouble doing it. Then we quickly realize its importance in maintaining our comfortable functioning.

Research has consistently demonstrated that rapid eye movement (REM), also known as dream sleep, helps us maintain our comfort and sanity. People deprived of that in the laboratory for a couple of days literally experience a synthetic psychosis that disappears as soon as they are allowed to dream. People wrestling with anxiety or depression report much stronger symptoms when they haven't had a good night's sleep. Even those without such problems or symptoms drag sluggishly along when their sleep is limited or interrupted.

The same is true in Cancerville. Staring at the ceiling above your bed in the middle of the night does little to recharge your batteries; it is like forgetting to plug in your cell phone. Insomnia, in any form, prevents your dam from receiving a sufficient energy boost. Let's use my model of the mind to understand the important role sleep plays in your day-to-day functioning.

When you go to sleep, so does your dam. It has been working hard all day, is damn tired, and needs to be recharged. While it sleeps, cess is released all over your head. We call the results dreaming. This is why dreams can be so confusing when remembered, as they contain pieces of yesterday and from a while ago, all connected like an abstract, avant-garde movie.

Freud called dreams "the royal road to the unconscious." He felt he could understand what was going on in his patient's unconscious mind if he could interpret the symbolic message embedded in the dream. This may be true sometimes, but in my opinion, the importance of sleep is that cess is being discharged and vented, while dams are being recharged in preparation for tomorrow. This is why when you don't sleep well, you don't feel or function very well the next day.

The various relaxation activities and exercises that I have described can all contribute to a more nourishing night's sleep. They allow your mind to wind down. They induce the kind of brain rhythms that allow you to peacefully fall off to sleep and remain asleep. They literally help turn down your mind and shut down any rumination, which is especially helpful in Cancerville.

I Can't Call This One a Tool

For many people, prayer serves as a calming, relaxing, and inspirational experience. Not only does it connect them to a power greater than themselves, but it also can induce a calming, trance-like state. The nice thing about prayer is that it is portable. You don't have to be in a church or temple to draw strength from it. One can pray anywhere, anytime, and in any way.

In addition, studies have shown that seriously ill people who had others praying for them had a higher survival rate than those for whom no prayers were offered. This was true whether or not the patients were aware that people were praying. Yet independent of those findings, if prayer helps you in calming, healing, and empowering ways, then I encourage you to do just that every day or several times a day for that matter.

In addition, if a symbol of faith or hope can help you feel more empowered, I encourage you to place it in your home, wear it, or carry it in your purse or briefcase. In Cancerville, even something as simple as a rubber band with meaningful words inscribed on it seems to help people feel more powerful and hopeful. That is why I offer a complimentary purple wristband with the statement "DAM STRONG!" with each order at www.cancerville.com.

In Sum

As I type these words, the enormous fiord-based mountains, which are warmly blanketed by layers of low-lying clouds, are still here to provide peaceful and relaxing sensory images for me. I do periodically look up from the keyboard. Though the day may be steely gray, reminding me of the one at Sloan-Kettering, my feelings are lighter and brighter. This is in part because we are, literally and figuratively, distanced from Cancerville. In addition, my already relaxed feelings have been significantly enhanced by the calming influence of these majestic images that I will long remember.

I hope that in Cancerville you will seek out calming sensory experiences from time to time. It certainly doesn't require a trip across the world. You can purchase a CD or DVD, or you can take advantage of free relaxation materials over the Internet; these can be very helpful to you at this agitating time. My biased view is that it is very important that you find that which helps you relax and/or distracts you from Cancerville and commit to engage whenever you can.

Now, let us turn to other user-friendly tools that help modify negative and uncomfortable thoughts. Negativity in Cancerville can take away from your hopefulness and positive self-talk. To tend to this demanding land, you need to be able to influence and take charge of your thoughts and resulting feelings by nudging them toward a more neutral or even positive direction.

CHAPTER 16

I will try to choose what I think about each day.

Cognitive Tools for Taking Charge of Your Mind

I have stressed the importance of maintaining hopeful and positive thoughts and self-talk in the chapters dealing with realistic optimism as well as positive self-talk. The question remains how to help you get there when you are wrestling with all of the difficulties and negativity that Cancerville can present.

Most people are prone to ruminate on issues that upset them in all areas of their lives. When your loved one is in Cancerville, all of that pressure, worry, and concern becomes a major obsessional flood; it is hard to think about anything else. Cancerville shouts at us from a "bully pulpit." I hope the cognitive tools I will share with you in this chapter, as well as everything else we discuss, will help you shout back even louder.

These simple tools will help you keep your mind stronger, balanced, and more able to support your trying Cancerville experience. They will strengthen your dam as you care for and help your loved one. Combining these cognitive tools with the relaxation ones described in the previous chapter can make for a powerful and protective support net.

We All Have the Same Architecture—More or Less

When I look back over my shoulder at the many people I have talked to and helped in my office for all these years, I clearly see some patterns that have occurred over and over again. We all have the same architecture, as reflected in my model of the mind, even though we are all unique individuals. What vary from person to person are our genes and scenes. Our genome and the contents of our life experiences, which account for our individual natures, are as unique as our fingerprints.

In my opinion, magnificent as our brains and minds are, the design could have been improved upon by the addition of some more direct vents to eliminate cess. Had they asked me, I would have definitely suggested some modifications along the lines of how our bodies eliminate waste. But hey, I never got the email; I wasn't even on the committee. However, the tools in this chapter and the previous one help minimize our cess and keep it from building up.

Please understand that I did not invent the cognitive tools I will be describing, although I did rename them for this book. Also, know that not all of these tools work for everyone and not all tools work all of the time. It is a little like going to the gym for a workout. You won't like or use every piece of equipment, but the more you use a few of these mind-muscle builders, the stronger and more resilient you and your mind will become.

Changing the Channel

Our minds are like TV screens and your challenge is to find the remote; don't even bother looking under the couch pillows. Once you do find and practice using it, you can move the channel to a calmer mental "movie" if your mind wanders into negative spaces.

A Future Movie

For example, it is helpful to picture a time in the future when life will be better, your loved one is safe, and your lives are back to everyday living. Picture his or her hair having grown back, having put back the weight lost in Cancerville, or having lost the puffiness that some of the meds can cause.

In this regard, I encouraged Rob to try to visualize in his mind's eye being back on the ice at the hockey rink with both of his sons. Time on the rink hasn't happened yet, but I am optimistic that it will; time on the baseball diamond happened this summer.

In November, I also encouraged Rob to picture his son and wife being home from Sloan-Kettering for Christmas. As you already know, under the stressful conditions of Cancerville, minds can go back and forth. After my encouragement, Rob could happily picture his family being together at Christmas, but then think, "OMG, what if it doesn't happen? What if my son is still in the hospital?" This would immediately eliminate and undo the optimistic image and take him right back to negative space.

I suggested that he assume his homecoming would happen and realize that if it didn't, it would not be terrible. It might put a damper on Christmas 2010, but then his happy family homecoming image could shift to Easter and Christmas 2011. Or he could picture having Christmas in January or whenever his son came home. Many soldiers have delayed holidays, birthdays, or anniversaries, as they usually can't get home on cue. The same applies to the "soldiers" of Cancerville.

Rob's family was, in fact, back home in time for a happy and heartfelt Christmas morning. There was no greater or more meaningful gift that day than their being reunited and together. Truth!

A Past Movie

Another useful channel changer, if your mind becomes overwhelmed with negativity, is to replay a pleasant, positive scene from your past, possibly involving your loved one. You can draw upon your built-in DVD or DVR player to watch it all again. I can recall watching happy family scenes on my personal TV during Jodi's treatment time in Cancerville. It was easy to visualize her arrival day from Korea, her Bat Mitzvah, her dance performances, and many other happy scenes.

You can also draw upon pleasant images unrelated to your loved one. When I sat in the waiting room at Sloan-Kettering, I closed my eyes and traveled somewhere else in my mind's eye. I put myself on my favorite beach in Jupiter, Florida, where I watched the edge of the sea kissing the sand as birds flew by against the backdrop of blue skies and billowy clouds.

The faster you mentally leave an unpleasant scene by creating different images, the calmer you can become. The beauty of my mind and yours is its versatility. There are more soothing images you can play on your personal TV than there are channels on deluxe cable TV. Use those to your advantage when your mind "freezes" in the cesspool of Cancerville or, for that matter, becomes stuck in any other muck life throws in your direction.

You have some choice in the pictures you play on your personal TV just as you decide which pictures to rent and watch on your home TV. When you can, try to watch some "happily ever after" movies in your head, just like the Hollywood of old regularly produced. When you need to change the channel, know that you are able to accomplish that very result when you put your mind to it.

Obviously, there will be times in Cancerville when "escaping" in this way is not advisable or possible. For example, I do not encourage you to change the channel in the middle of a tense doctor meeting. However, once it is over and you are back home, more peaceful images may just help calm your mind and move it to more positive self-talk.

Fantasies are Free

Fantasies can take changing the channel to a whole new level of creativity. You can enjoy a fantasy just about anytime or anywhere. Fantasies occur when our minds make a movie about an enjoyable but unlikely event. It is about letting your mind roam freely into any area that you like. People fantasize about being the CEO of a major corporation, the President of the United States, a lotto winner, a beauty queen, or a stud muffin. As I said, fantasies are free. This is true as long as you keep them in your mind. Once you start emailing, texting, or tweeting, watch out as they can easily become very costly.

You can be the producer, director, and star all at the same time and see whatever images you want. Reality has nothing to do with it. Your creative mind can picture anything that serves to comfort, relax, or distract you. Fantasy is a powerful tool to create prettier pictures than the ones you may be dealing with in real life.

I'm not telling you anything you don't already know. You have probably had thousands of daydreams and fantasies since you were a youngster. What I am simply encouraging you to do is go there intentionally at appropriate times when your mind is rumbling like a volcano ready to blow. Feel free to try it and see if you can make it work for you.

Whatever fantasies you create need to be dam building. For example, see yourself writing the next blockbuster book about your favorite hobby or whatever interests you. See yourself getting an award or doing something courageous or important.

Picture your garden weedless and in full bloom. The point is that fantasies are truly free and can occasionally free you from the heavy burdens with which you are dealing.

Sometimes fantasies can even be a source of inspiration. Remember the one I chose to use in order to write this book in a clear and strong way—"That ball is going, going, and it's gone!"

The D That Comes After ABC

In Chapter 11, "The Power of Positive Self-Talk," I spoke about the ABCs created by Dr. Ellis and his cognitive colleagues. As you recall, A is for an adverse activating event, B for beliefs triggered by the event, and C for the emotional consequences caused by the belief. In this cognitive model, D stands for disputing the belief. We previously contrasted the way pessimists and optimists approach Cancerville using the ABC model. Let's review this again:

The pessimist says…

A: My loved one has cancer.
B: My loved one will not survive.
C: I feel depressed, terrified, anxious, and overwhelmed. I can't deal with this.

The optimist says …

A: My loved one has cancer.
B: Many people survive these days.
C: Although I am not happy we are here, I am hopeful we will get through it together. I will do all I can to be helpful and supportive.

As I have previously said, my encouragement towards optimism needs to be realistic. There is an obvious and significant difference between a pessimist and someone whose loved one's cancer is Stage IV, has seriously metastasized, or is unresponsive to chemo. The degree to which you can dispute your negative beliefs is directly related to your loved one's situation; ultimately, those realities must be taken into account.

Cognitive psychologists have found that people can be taught and encouraged to dispute their automatic negative beliefs and move to more positive or at least neutral thoughts. This often demands that we replace those beliefs with ones that are more comfortable, acceptable, and tolerable. In the previous example, the pessimist needs to dispute his or her catastrophic belief because it can rapidly cause an emotional meltdown. As soon as a shift is made to the more hopeful belief, the emotional tone and reaction change, and the person can move forward.

To dispute your negative beliefs, you need to think and act like a savvy defense attorney. Think of how the famous ones are able to spin potentially damaging evidence against their client in ways that neutralize or even reverse it. Appeal to the "jury" of your mind to allow for alternative beliefs, explanations, and rationales. Be convincing and creative in reprocessing upsetting ideas that will only take you to dark and scary places. Dispute them in every way you can to change and reframe your belief and the resulting emotions. Remember Benje's story in Chapter 4—"At least Jodi has a chance, a good chance." And he was undeniably correct.

For example, let's dispute the pessimist's belief that "My loved one will not survive." Here is my disputational dissertation to the jury of your mind:

> Try hard not to be pessimistic, ladies and gentlemen of the jury. We have strong and consis-tent evidence that, thanks to marvelous medical progress these days, many people survive their Cancerville experience—almost two-thirds become survivors. We have many reasons to be optimistic.

Innovations occur regularly and reliably. For example, the many types of targeted treatments, including those delivered by interventional radiologists, are already being used in effective ways. These provide direct treatment of cancer without many of the unpleasant side effects. Gene studies hold great promise in more specifically matching specific cancer types to targeted treatments. Who knows what other advances will be coming soon? I am betting on more and more progress. You need to try to do that as well.

My belief in progress is based upon the adage that the past is often an excellent predictor of the future. We have seen devastating diseases such as smallpox, scarlet fever, and polio completely eliminated by the scientific progress of vaccines. In 1952, the year I turned ten, over fifty thousand people were diagnosed with polio in the United States, including a teen who lived on the first floor of my apartment building. Public swimming pools were closed, people avoided large crowds, and parents—especially mine—were frantic. In 2002, the number of diagnosed cases of polio in the United States was zero! Every year, I believe, we get a little closer to eliminating cancer from our world too.

In the meantime, ladies and gentlemen of the jury, you already know the dedication of your medical team of doctors, nurses, and other professionals. They may keep you waiting, but not wanting. They want to win as much as you do. I dispute your assumption and choose to see things more optimistically. You need to agree and see things my way by finding in favor of your

> loved one's survival. I rest my case and hope it helps you "rest" just a little easier!

I hope this helps you to dispute any negativity that your mind generates and increases your hopefulness and optimism about your loved one's outcome in Cancerville.

I also believe that there is a D in my model. It stands for: "DAM STRONG!" power. As we now know, it is our cess that causes us to catastrophize and remain stuck, as if by crazy glue, to pessimistic beliefs. It is our dam that helps us dispute this negativity and reverse it, which allows for realistic optimism and positive self-talk. These, in turn, allow us much calmer and hopeful feelings.

Since no one knows or can predict the future, assume it to be a positive one for your loved one and yourself; try not to allow negativity to creep into your mind. If you have a pessimistic belief, use your dam to dispute it as strongly as you can. Whether you have a law degree or not does not matter. What matters are the challenges and disputations you submit on your own behalf.

Putting it Away

This tool works for some but not for others. Hard as they might try, some people just can't put their worries away, even overnight. They tend to stick to them as if held in place by cement. Still, I encourage you to give this tool a try and see if you can make it work.

Sometimes, the best thing to do with your worries and ruminating thoughts is to shelve them. Imagine that it is 2 a.m. and you can't sleep. Your mind is running wild with fear, yet you need to get up in a few hours for your loved one's chemo appointment. Say to yourself: "Self, we are going to take all of my fears and worries and put them on a shelf in the bathroom. I can pick them up in the morning or after I get back home tomorrow, if I so choose. But for now, they will wait so I can get some sleep."

Alternately, you can try to put them into storage for a longer period of time. In this case, the self-speech is slightly different: "I'm not getting anywhere with all these annoying thoughts; I'm just making myself more 'crazy' than I already am. I am going to put these in a box on a shelf in my closet, and try my best to let them stay there. They are not helping me one bit."

In addition to these useful delays in your worries, some people draw upon their spiritual beliefs to help them cope better. They send off their concerns and worries to God instead of to a shelf, carton, or other storage area. This, no doubt, is where the expression "Let go and let God" comes from. In so doing, these people are placing their faith in a higher power and praying for a positive result. They are also delegating their worry to a spiritual force greater than themselves. They clear their mind in this way and are, hopefully, better able to get to sleep. Try to push away your worries and other negative thoughts whenever and however you can.

Using the Brake, Not the Gas

Beyond the power of positive self-talk, there is power in any self-talk that encourages your mind to stop spewing cess all over your head. This tool encourages you to talk back to your mind in ways that try to stop such disruptive thoughts and beliefs.

When these occur, just say: "Please stop now," or just "Stop" a couple of times. As you say those words, picture a red stop sign in your mind. See yourself stopping your car for that sign, and as you slowly put on the brake in this image, imagine you are doing the same thing in your mind so that your thoughts and feelings can move on to more positive and productive subjects. Some people find it helpful to wear a rubber band (with or without a message) that they can snap to remind them to shut off negative inner thoughts that can pop up like weeds in the summer heat.

People often combine this practice with one of the other tools mentioned in this chapter or the previous one and find the blend of two or more quite helpful. For example, they get themselves into a calmer state through a relaxation exercise, and then picture the stop sign that helps them control and halt their ruminating thoughts. Or they see the stop sign, change the channel, and use a relaxation exercise to calm themselves. I encourage you to experiment and be creative. There are no hard and fast rules. There are just opportunities to take charge of your mind so that you can avoid being flooded with cess.

Wide Angle or Telephoto Lensing

Considering what our eyes choose to see and "film," they are amazing still and video cameras. Right now, I am looking at the last sentence on my computer screen and can see it completely. If I want, however, I can choose to focus on the word "cameras" and make all other words go blurry. Or I can stare at the sentence and allow my peripheral vision to see the bulletin board of pictures above my desk, the printer to my right, and the plants and sunshine on the patio to my left. My eyes and yours have quite an impressive set of lenses.

How we use these lenses is what creates the proverbial glass half full or half empty perspective. I can choose to focus on the debris and the large layers of seaweed that occasionally invade the ocean at the beach in Jupiter. Or I can focus on the blue sky, large white clouds, gentle waves as they hit the shore, and the lovely birds searching for their targets down below the waterline. These impressive images make the debris and seaweed meaningless.

I had similar choices in Cancerville, and so do you. I could have focused on the pain that Jodi was going through, but instead I pushed myself to see her gain there. For example, I could have seen and snapped a "picture" of the harsh chemicals going into her veins on those difficult days, but I fought hard to try to use my telephoto lens and see those bloody bastard cells being destroyed, hundreds at a time, like a powerful B52 bomb strike. It took me a while to adjust my zoom and my words, but I am confident that you can do that too.

As another example, I could have seen Jodi's bald head through my internal camera and felt sad and down; but I chose wide-angle and saw that she was still a beautiful young woman, even without hair. This lens enabled me to see that we are not defined by our hair, or other superficial characteristics. As I pictured all of Jodi's special qualities, I paired those images with the thought that "hair grows back," and left her baldness behind. By modifying and altering what my eyes chose to see and my mind thought, I could literally change my beliefs and move my feelings in a positive direction. In this simple but powerful way, so can you!

In Sum

It is not easy to avoid the challenging, and at times mind-boggling, thoughts and feelings that come along with Cancerville. These are, unfortunately, just part of the nature of the territory. There are, however, many ways to let go of these negative thoughts and convert them to ones that allow for inspiration instead of perspiration. The above tools represent different strategies you can use to take charge of your mind and actively work to move it from negative to more positive thoughts and self-talk. By using these tools, you may be able to bypass cess that adds to your pool, erodes your dam, and is agitating and counterproductive.

You can experiment and try to tailor these tools to fit your needs and mindset. When it comes to matters of the mind, there is much room for your own personal creativity. Combining these tools with those of the previous chapter can make for a powerful antidote to help counter negativity.

Often, a mental health counselor or support group can help you learn to use and apply the tools I have described or others that are similar. This personal approach to drawing upon cognitive tools is only one of the many helpful benefits of having such support in your corner. Let's talk more about these valuable resources in the following chapter.

CHAPTER 17

I will seek support if and when I need it.

Having a Counselor and/or Support Group in Your Corner

Much like a nutritionist promoting veggies and vitamins or a dental hygienist promoting flossing, I am biased about the importance of mental health counseling as a worthwhile coping, balancing, and healthy living tool. This is true in everyday life, but even more so when dealing with Cancerville. Very few things are more powerful than one person supportively helping another get through a difficult time. I say this based on having helped many people in my career and having been helped personally as well.

A Shrink Will Help You Grow

In my book *Getting Back Up From an Emotional Down,* one of the chapters is called "Everyone Needs a Shrink I Think." That was my belief in the late 1980s and remains so now. Generally speaking, cess builds up over time while dams erode. Thus, as time goes on, many people struggle with a variety of emotional discomforts and disorders that include anxiety, depression, low self-esteem, guilt, food-related problems, other addictions, and the like.

This is precisely why millions are on psychiatric meds and millions more need them. It is also why we have become gloppers who use a wide range of "pacifiers" to fill the voids in our lives. Too many walk weakly to the finish line, and a significant number of others crawl there on their bellies. "DAM STRONG!" is an empowering call to take better care of ourselves in and out of Cancerville.

If people can benefit from a counselor in their everyday lives, they certainly can use one while in Cancerville. The reasons are quite obvious. Cancerville's cess adds to already existing everyday cess in a way that makes for hurricane warnings, tornado watches, and major flooding. As we discussed in Part III, anxieties, anger, and guilt move rapidly into our cesspool and then to the surface of our mind, like a submarine coming up quickly from the ocean floor.

In Cancerville, your head can quickly become jammed, fogged, and almost numb with an overload of emotion. Like a boxer, you will try to shake off that shot to your head until the next left jab or right hook catches you off-guard and puts you even further off-balance. To counterbalance this, you can benefit from having someone in your corner who can help get you through this battle. He or she can't take the journey for you, but at least that person can help wipe the emotional sweat away. A professional can also help you apply the tools described in the previous two chapters and perhaps teach you some others, as well, while offering a safe place to vent feelings and receive support.

Resistance to Seeking Professional Help

Despite the value I see coming from counseling, many in Cancerville will still resist seeking out and drawing upon this type of assistance. Instead, they choose to go it alone or to rely on family and friends. Hopefully, those close to you are positive supports; however, they likely lack the skill, knowledge, expertise, or objectivity of a professional. Keep in mind that much of the advice you receive from others, well-meaning as it is intended to be, can turn out to be useless at best and hurtful at worst. This is my bias and frequent observation, but it is possible that you are fortunate and have special family members and/or friends who are good listeners and supportive people on your team.

A professionally trained psychiatrist, psychologist, therapist, social worker, or counselor may be much better positioned to be of help than a layperson. Moreover, it is helpful to take the dam supports you have been taught in your visit home with you, while leaving your cess on the floor of my office or those of my colleagues.

Notwithstanding all of my encouraging endorsements of therapy and counseling, people's resistance to that help has been well known since the time of Freud. Many have told me they would rather have a root canal without nerve gas or novocaine than come to my office. It wasn't about me, and I never took it personally, as I am an easygoing, pleasant, and supportive psychologist.

Resistance is about people not wanting to face themselves and their issues. Just as we don't like to look in the mirror if our bellies are too bloated, we don't like to see the bulging mess in our cesspools. Nor do we enjoy confronting our glopful habits that result from such cess. Most of us would much rather just continue with them, unhealthy as they might be. Sometimes, as I spoke about previously, denial can be healthy and helpful; other times it can be very destructive.

Another reason many people resist counseling is that they are private and feel more comfortable maintaining a low profile. They feel threatened when imagining sitting across from a stranger and speaking honestly and openly about their lives, their problems, and themselves. People generally tend to suppress and repress embarrassing and sensitive frustrations, fears, and feelings as a way to avoid dealing with and confronting them. The same is true of our secrets; we do not like to think about them, let alone talk about them openly.

Finally, there is a popular belief that often keeps people from seeking professional assistance. Many feel that they "should" handle their lives and their problems on their own; I warned you early on about the danger of "shoulds." Though mainly prevalent among men, I have met many women who feel the same way. Usually, these people have been taught this while growing up and have this mythological belief embedded strongly in their minds. This distorted belief takes independence and self-sufficiency to a very exaggerated level. I often say to such a person that seeing a counselor is no different from seeking medical or dental help. Surely, you would not expect to fill your own cavity; why then would you expect to be able to fill the holes in your dam on your own?

Thus, for a variety of personal reasons, many avoid seeking out counseling support. Oddly enough, they are often the people who could most benefit from this experience. I am hopeful that if you need it, you will push past your resistance and participate.

Sounds of Silence

As Paul Simon and Art Garfunkel taught us many years ago, as we began to awaken from the repressive 1950s, "Silence like a cancer grows." In these simple yet wise words, they summed up everything that is wrong with suppressing one's feelings in any emotionally charged situation. Silence fills pools and weakens dams. The more people "stuff" painful feelings, the more cesspools grow and the more these feelings come back to bite in one way or another. Emotional "malignancy" is also a debilitating, dangerous, and difficult disease to treat. Simon and Garfunkel were undeniably correct.

When people visiting my office talk, they are usually venting cess and unstuffing themselves. In that sense, counseling has the same cathartic value as a powerful enema. When I respond as an interactive counselor, I am helping to rebuild and strengthen dams by filling in some of the cracks and crevices that have developed over time.

I hope that while you are in Cancerville, your resistance to seeking counseling support will be diminished since you are not coming for an overall emotional tune-up or treatment for a specific psychiatric disorder. The focus is primarily on present day issues; you are not signing up to inspect the "dirty diapers" of your past.

It is not your general history that I would focus on if you were visiting my office for Cancerville support as much as your present circumstances, coping skills, health history, and concerns about your loved one's journey. My goal would be to provide individualized support based on the details of your situation. I would help you embrace realistic optimism and learn to use relaxing and cognitive tools tailored to your needs and nature. It would be a practical and personalized effort to help you cope better and maintain your own health and balance during this difficult time.

Warning Signs of Needing Additional Support

It is my bias and belief that just about everyone with a loved one in Cancerville can benefit from professional support. However, some situations are more demanding than others. Here are some warning signs and symptoms that suggest some immediate professional assistance could be beneficial:

- significant difficulty sleeping, eating, concentrating, and/or performing other basic life functions
- wide-ranging mood swings within short periods of time
- high anxiety for long periods of time or frequent panic attacks
- disabling depression, spending too much time in bed, and/or long-lasting tearfulness

- fighting constantly with everyone
- losing faith, hope, or the ability to be positive
- using glop regularly
- an inability to distract yourself, use the previously mentioned tools, or find a way to relax and calm down
- thoughts of hurting yourself in any way

Choosing a Helpful Professional

As with all professions, not all mental health counselors are created equal, although the majority are caring and capable people who are committed to the good of your cause. Choosing the right mental health counselor is a very important decision that is too often based upon issues that have nothing to do with the counselor's competence or your comfort. Both are key components for a helpful match with a mental health professional.

For example, people may choose a support professional solely because of the proximity to their home or office, whether the counselor participates in their health insurance program, or someone's recommendation. These practical issues make for a good starting point to one's search. In addition, however, a brief phone conversation or first visit meeting will help to determine if you are comfortable with the rapport and fit. It is important for you to find someone with whom you feel at ease and who you see as trustworthy.

Beyond seeking out someone with specific Cancerville experience, I encourage you to initially visit with a variety of questions in mind:

- Does this person seem sincerely interested in my situation or does it feel like a recorded announcement?
- Is there more emphasis placed on billing issues than on my issues?
- Did my appointment start close to the scheduled time?
- Do I feel comfortable and free to speak openly or do I feel judged and on guard?

- Do I feel I can trust this person?
- Is the setting comfortable and appropriate or am I jammed into a room that is too small, hot, or cold?
- Am I given undivided attention or are there phone or other interruptions?
- Am I given the full time I was promised?
- Is my visit helpful in setting some goals and offering me support and understanding?
- Did what he or she say make sense?

Hopefully, your experience with a counselor or therapist will go well. If it doesn't, please don't hesitate to try someone else. Choosing the right professional for you is a very important part of the process.

Support Groups

Not all people are comfortable with or can afford a one-on-one counseling experience. As I'm sure you know, there are many support group possibilities both in person and over the Internet. I have met many people for whom support groups were very helpful and some who had less than positive experiences. In most instances, our personal preferences determine the helpfulness and value of the experience. Potential benefits of any growth experience are limited by whether we feel comfortable there or not.

Though I have facilitated many types of support groups over the years, I was not eager to participate in one related to Cancerville. Ronnie "dragged" me to one meeting, but I did not like it; it did not help me, so I never went back. I probably needed to check out one or two others to see if I could find a group that was more comfortable and helpful for me.

Despite my reluctance, support groups at hospitals and at places like Gilda's Club, etc. serve a valuable purpose for many people. Certainly, keep your mind open to this option, and see if a support group can be worthwhile for you. Some people find it very advantageous to be able to call other group members when their feelings and moods shift with the Cancerville tides. An added advantage is that almost all support groups are free.

There are many cancer specific support groups, chat rooms, and bulletin boards on the Internet these days. They are worth a try as well, especially since they are easy and efficient to access. They also allow you to maintain your anonymity and only share that information with which you feel comfortable. In addition, you can choose to be an active or passive participant.

Support groups are also a helpful adjunct to individual counseling for some people. They report very different experiences in each and find the combination and synergy even more worthwhile.

In Sum

I strongly believe that counseling and/or a support group experience can be very helpful generally, and especially for those who have a loved one in Cancerville. My bias, however, need not be your command, as I understand that these experiences are not for everyone. I fully respect your right to decline.

My hope is that this book provides a valuable support to help you cope better with your Cancerville experience. No book, however, can replace an individual, tailored counseling experience or being part of an ongoing support group. I hope you will keep an open mind and will consider the possibility of these resources. I know individual counseling helped me personally, and I believe it can be helpful to you and many other people as well.

Crying is an important and healthy emotional vent at difficult or joyous times in our lives. Let's discuss this in more detail in the next chapter.

CHAPTER 18

Crying at times is okay.

Big Boys and Girls Do Cry

It is likely that you will cry when your loved one is in Cancerville, as cancer has a way of bringing even the strongest people to their emotional knees. But that is okay; crying is actually helpful. It goes without saying that Ronnie and I cried many times in Cancerville, but we always worked our way back to a more comfortable and clear-headed position.

Most of us are able to maintain a stiff upper lip until we get to a private or safe place where we feel more comfortable allowing our tears to flow. I always say that tissues are the most costly part of my overhead. That's not exactly true, but many do feel safe crying in their therapist or counselor's office. That is a really helpful vent and a place where those feelings can be left behind. Take the dam builders with you and leave your cess under my area rug. The cleaning crew will take care of the rest later.

Often, I will ask the person I am helping what his or her tears are "saying" to gain a clearer understanding of their deeper meaning. Almost always, people are able to identify the thoughts and feelings that triggered them. In my opinion, there are many different feelings that can cause us to cry. I believe that tears are a form of wordless communication that represents a variety of emotions.

Where it All Began

From our very beginnings, crying serves a variety of useful purposes. As infants, it is our only communication device to signal discomfort. It is our emergency call as helpless babies, that shout-out to our caretakers that we are hungry, tired, have a dirty diaper, or need a big burp or an even bigger hug. An infant's tears come from irritating or painful physical sensations, since their thoughts and emotions have yet to develop.

Crying is also a vent that lasts long after infancy to both express and flush out our child or teen-based displeasures and emotional wounds. Our hurts, disappointments, social rejections, academic failures, losses, sibling assaults, and other abuses all flow out in a tantrum of tears.

As adults, we still cry from strong physical pains, but our thoughts and feelings are more likely to be the stimulus for our tears. For example, we think about our loved one's distress, feel very sad/bad/mad, and our adult self, filled with loving concern, can lead us down a tearful path. There, our pained adult parts may meet up with the little boy or girl who lives within our grown and aging self. This is precisely why big boys and girls do cry in and out of Cancerville.

For those who feel crying reflects weakness, you need only look to the many settings outside of Cancerville where it is perfectly appropriate and acceptable for adults to cry. Emotional movies, celebrations, award ceremonies, and many other situations all cause people to cry freely without being self-conscious or judged as weak. Think about the big brawny athletes whose tear-filled towels appear randomly at the conclusion of the "big game." Both the winners and the losers shed their share of tears. These tears come about from the overwhelming ecstasy of winning or the gut-wrenching agony of defeat.

In her book *It's Always Personal*,[15] Anne Kreamer talks about the value of people crying in the workplace. She says, "Crying at work is transformative and can open the door to change." Certainly, if people can comfortably cry in these different situations without embarrassment, you can cry Cancerville tears too.

As we already know, Cancerville creates many intense feelings, some of which can trigger our tears. As I mentioned, I believe there are different types of tears that are based upon and represent different thoughts and feelings. Knowing about them will help you more clearly understand what you are feeling and dealing with when your tears flow in Cancerville.

Tears of Shock and Awful

Ronnie's phone call alerting me to Jodi's diagnosis was a tear-filled explosion. Her tears spoke the otherwise unspeakable devastation of a mom whose world had just come crashing down on her head with the terrifying and overwhelming force of an emotional earthquake. Every single word of that brief conversation was streaked, if not flooded, with her tears.

I concluded my session with the client sitting across from me in mid-sentence and came right home. That was only the second time in my practice that I did that; the previous time was also for a serious family emergency. The twenty-minute ride home seemed like an eternity and yet much too short a time to face a pain-filled reality.

Upon arriving home, Ronnie and I both cried for a while until we could calm ourselves. Once we regained our composure, we called Jodi. Even though Ronnie and I were feeling worse than terrible, we were able to plant some small positive seeds into some pretty dark soil in our daughter's mind. Obviously, she was quite shaken after receiving a terrifying and overwhelming diagnosis.

Ultimately, those seeds took root and helped her already strong nature grow into beanstalks of hope and optimism. I believe that her positive expectations contributed to her recovery. I have always felt, both in my practice and in my life, that it is never too early to plant a seed—beanstalks do take time to grow.

Tears of Inequity

Considering the stakes and pressures, as well as your loved one's suffering, you have every right to shed some tears of inequity from time to time and vent your fury at the unfairness of it all. In this context, to not do that seems less than appropriate.

When your loved one is in Cancerville, you stand in the proverbial Job-like position asking, "Why us God?" When no clear answer comes, tears over this undeniable inequity often do. You might want to read Rabbi Harold Kushner's view on this complex subject. After his young son died of a dread disease unrelated to Cancerville, he wrote *When Bad Things Happen to Good People*.[16] You need not be Jewish to relate.

As you know from the Introduction, my "This cannot be my daughter's turn!" lament and associated tears were all about the unfairness of Cancerville. It is undeniably a difficult hand to be dealt, but as I have stressed throughout, it is all about playing a difficult hand as well as we can. Actions and distractions help us look away from the unfairness of it all.

Tears of Sadness

Cancerville is a place that promotes sadness. How can you not be sad that your loved one is there and being forced to deal with all of its challenges and demands? Similarly, how can you not be sad that you are there as well? Few places can be as hurtful to your loved one and you as Cancerville. Fortunately, the majority will get through it and can slowly return to a calmer life. Let us assume for now that your loved one will too.

When you are sad, your tears are a natural response and release. They wash away some of your painful feelings and allow you to return to a more comfortable position so you can focus on the progress that is being made. Being sad, in and out of Cancerville, is natural—so is crying from time to time when you are sad.

I worked very hard to shake the sad feelings that would sweep over me like a cold gust of Chicago wind in February. I kept putting on the emotional equivalent of a heavy winter coat, complete with scarf and mittens. That is definitely not easy for a guy from Fort Lauderdale. Despite drawing upon the tools I have described, feeling sad caused tears to fall from time to time. They were a helpful vent and enabled us to cope better.

Even now, all these years later, as we read and edit certain parts of this book, Ronnie and I still shed sad tears that drip slowly down our cheeks and dampen the pages. We take a break, catch our breath, and return to our work. These tears help us vent the cess related to those painful memories and allow us to just move forward! No matter how positive your loved one's outcome, Cancerville leaves a residue of sadness that doesn't really ever go away. How could it?

Tears of the Unknown

As I have previously mentioned, you probably are not comfortable with the unknown. You, like almost all people, feel much better when you think and feel you are in control. Whether you truly are in control or have just built an illusion of control is not what matters. The problem is that in Cancerville there is no way to keep the illusion going; Cancerville and certainty do not typically co-exist.

I fully understand crying about unknown possibilities, but I discourage you from dwelling on that for very long. As I repeatedly reminded myself, it is not just in Cancerville that you don't know what's coming around the corner. The unknown is scary all over the place simply because you know, all too well, that you don't know! So just as you probably don't worry and cry about other possible unknown outcomes outside of Cancerville, I urge you to cry briefly, vent your feelings, and then refocus on positive outcomes for your loved one.

Tears of Commiseration

The question can be raised as to whether it is appropriate or not to cry in front of or with your loved one. There is no clear answer that will fit all situations or all people. I believe the answer is similar to the one we discussed in Chapter 11 when we talked about authentic versus artificial communication. You will recall that Dr. Coyne talked about "protective buffering" and the division among professionals on this topic. The examples that I suggested were more balanced and avoided going to one extreme or the other.

I hope you can strike a balance that allows for support and hopefulness as well as expressing your genuine feelings, including tears. Your tears may or may not flow when your loved ones' are flowing. It may occur naturally or you may choose to suppress them. It is a very personal issue and may or may not be a conscious choice.

Would I encourage you to cry hysterically for fifteen or twenty minutes in your loved one's presence? If I could write the script, I would try to contain such scenes to a few moments of a tear-filled embrace. That said, however, there is no faucet connected to our tear ducts. I encourage you to do as you and your mind and body need.

Let's keep in mind that since crying is a healthy vent and release, modeling that for your loved one is helpful. Of course, these words need to be tempered by the age of your loved one. If it is a child who has never seen you cry, I encourage a much stiffer upper lip and a more private venting. If your loved one is an adult and you cry in his or her presence, try to return quickly to more neutral or positive and hopeful positions. "We will get through this," "I believe you will be okay," or "Let's put our faith and trust in God," are all helpful post-cry affirming comments.

I don't recall us crying with Jodi or she in front of us other than on her walk to the OR. We all cried privately, as is our nature. Our inner programs guide us automatically, especially in our more sensitive zones. Once again, I remind you that there is no "right" way; there is only your way and what feels comfortable to you.

Invisible Tears

There is another form of tears that I discovered in Cancerville. I came to call them invisible tears. These occurred when no one knew that I was crying except me—but I was. These tears flowed silently from my heart. They poured out with the force of a flood, and yet they went nowhere. There was no evidence of their existence because they stayed hidden inside me.

These invisible tears came in a variety of settings and from a variety of triggers. It was as simple as a newspaper article or as complicated as a visit to one of Jodi's doctors. It was a totally unrelated movie or show or a fleeting thought racing through my mind to nowhere in particular. In fact, all these years later, my invisible tears still flow from time to time. As I previously said, when I reread parts of this manuscript, both visible and invisible tears come on quietly but heavily. Many references take me right back to exceptionally difficult and dark days for Jodi, our family, and for me.

The problem with invisible tears is that instead of relieving your system by venting, they clog it further by tormenting. They leave an emotional residue that remains attached to your heart like the toxins of a cigarette or fatty deposits from a delicious but unhealthy plate of pâté. This is why it is helpful to cry visible tears to vent those invisible ones that can so easily stain the lining of your heart. Such stains leave you feeling down and sapped of energy and optimism. I truly believe crying can help protect your health as well as your mind. That is one of many reasons I allowed my tears to flow the night my friend Phil emailed me about his grandson having leukemia.

You may wonder why I said that crying could protect your body. It is the stress of suppressing painful feelings that concerns me. Such stress taxes your entire system. It compromises your immune system and your important organs. It weighs heavily on your body as well as your mind. It weakens you in every way. I simply want you to go through Cancerville as physically and emotionally strong as you possibly can. Crying from time to time will help you do just that.

Happy Tears

There are also tears of joy, happiness, and relief. These, of course, are the very best tears to experience. The winners of a sporting event or award, or people who cry at weddings and other celebrations, are feeling excited and elated. In *Getting Back Up From an Emotional Down*, I wrote, "When the dam laughs at the pool it often comes out in the form of a teardrop." Simply put, nothing feels quite so good as a prideful or joyous time when a dam deposit overrides a cess-based issue or worry.

These same happy feelings will occur when you receive good news about your loved one from the not-so-grim doctors. They can smile and really do enjoy positive news too. Just ask Rob how the meeting went when they excitedly announced they were finally ready to do the bone marrow transplant from one of his twins to the other.

Your tears after such a happening will be of a "thank goodness" kind. Such moments tenderly reinforce the positive thinking that I am encouraging. Savor these high-five moments and the tears that may flow because they are so very special.

I have always "enjoyed," in a bittersweet way, the feeling of happy and joyous tears. I cried them when I pulled to the side of I-95 as we drove back from Miami International Airport the day Jodi arrived from Korea to join our family. It was such a magical moment for all of us. I cried happy but invisible tears at her Bat Mitzvah as our beautiful Asian daughter chanted her prayers with the grace and ease of a rabbi. Of course, I cried at her Modern Day Fairy Tale, which I will share very, very soon.

There were similar tears of joy for the birth of and the high points of my sons' and grandsons' lives. There are times when the events in the lives of your loved ones overwhelm you with emotion. Love, in my opinion, is the most powerful of all of our emotions and leaves us vulnerable and sensitive to the highs and lows of the lives of our loved ones.

In Sum

Simply said, it is okay for adults to cry. Cancerville is an experience that absolutely demands tear-filled releases. These releases will help ease the emotional and physical pressures that build up on a daily basis.

I want you to feel okay with crying because, contrary to the popular belief that adults should just suck it up, big boys and girls do cry for a variety of reasons throughout their lives. My sincere hope is that the majority of your tears will be of the happy kind and will be commingled with laughter.

Laughter is the subject of the next chapter. Your immediate reaction may be that laughter and Cancerville do not belong in the same sentence. That was Ronnie's initial reaction too.

CHAPTER 19

I will find reasons to laugh from time to time.

Laughter in Cancerville

My goal in the previous chapter was to explain the importance of crying in Cancerville at times. I am hopeful that you will give yourself permission to do just that. I now want to encourage you to laugh there too.

I have included this chapter despite Ronnie's initial discouragement. She felt that the words cancer and laughter did not belong in the same sentence. You, like Ronnie, may wonder why I have included a chapter on laughter in a book about coping in Cancerville.

While I agree that cancer and Cancerville are not laughing matters, laughing matters a great deal when dealing with any serious illness or major life problem. Let me help you understand why I believe this is true. I hope that this will make it easier for you to see and believe in the potential helpfulness of laughter.

Obviously, Cancerville is a very serious place. That being said, funny and laughable things will happen there. Try not to be afraid of laughing at them, and don't stop yourself from cracking a joke or cracking up. Both you and your loved one can benefit from the tension release and venting power of laughter. As we shall soon see, the benefits can be richly rewarding.

Why Laughing Matters

I understand that laughing in Cancerville does not seem to fit the scene anymore than doing that in church or temple. Truth be known, it is okay to laugh in solemn places; the key is all in the timing and appropriateness. Recently, I was at a Catholic funeral where the priest said several humorous things about the deceased. We all laughed and enjoyed the pleasant memories as well as the tension release.

Making people laugh, especially those with heavy hearts, is a definite pride bank deposit for me. It is also a strategic part of my treatment plan. Yet it is always a judgment call, especially in Cancerville. These are sensitive times and your humor needs to be appropriate. Think about the fact that the late night comedians didn't air for a while post 9/11. Nothing they could have said would have worked, so they were smart enough to take a step back. We need to be that savvy and sensitive in Cancerville as well. When you are in doubt, leave it out.

Ronnie's memories of being in Cancerville are sad, pain-filled, and grim, as are mine. I also, however, remember laughing there at certain times. We sought out lighthearted and humorous plays and movies while in New York with Jodi and Zev. Being the good-humored man that I am, I continued, appropriately and respectfully, to facilitate laughter within my family, just as I do in my office. Jodi appears to have "inherited" my sense of humor and drew upon it frequently while going through Cancerville. Her lighter side definitely contributed to our brighter side; in fact, it still does! She and Zev arrived this morning for a visit and her texts had us laughing even before we reached the airport to pick them up.

Rob saw and chuckled at the humor of his inadvertently getting into a Jewish Sabbath elevator at Sloan-Kettering on a Saturday morning. Eager to see his son, he was frustrated that the elevator stopped on each floor. Being an Italian Catholic, it took him a moment to realize that very religious Jews don't "work" on the Sabbath, which includes not pressing buttons or turning on lights. So the elevator is programmed on Friday nights and Saturdays to stop at every floor. Laughing in that circumstance was much better than screaming, cursing, or calling himself or the elevator names.

Because of the value of a smile, giggle, chuckle, or belly laugh, I have tried to inject some humor into this less than funny book; I wanted to try to counterbalance the more difficult parts. I believe that humor is a salve that soothes raw nerve endings and minds flooded with cess.

Personal Experiences with Laughter

Much evidence, both anecdotal and research-based, has shown the positive influences of laughter. I need look no further than my Mom who laughed her way to over one hundred years of age. She validated all of the research studies that show a link between laughter and longevity. In a family not known for living longer than their early sixties, that was quite an accomplishment.

Mom laughed all the time at things she herself said. Many didn't seem humorous to me, but they must have tickled her funny bone in some magical way. Even when experiencing serious dementia toward the end of her life, she managed to laugh at different times. Though her life was pockmarked with tragedies and losses of all kinds, she counterbalanced that pain-filled cess with giggling and laughing dam supports.

I previously quoted Norman Cousins' groundbreaking book, *Anatomy of an Illness as Perceived by the Patient*. He described how he faced a serious, life-threatening disease, a degenerative condition of the spine that I can't even pronounce, let alone spell. He was told that his chances for a full recovery were one in five hundred. Upon hearing these long shot odds, Cousins stated, "It seemed clear to me that if I was to be that one in five hundred I had better be something more than a passive observer." These are obviously good words for people in Cancerville too.

Cousins took a variety of actions, any one of which could have made the ultimate difference, as he did eventually recover. He moved out of a hospital and into a hotel. He hired round the clock nurses to help him. He exposed himself to laughter by intentionally watching funny TV shows and movies and having his nurses read humorous books to him.

In addition, he had his doctor do blood work after his laughing sessions to measure his body's ability to fight off infection. The results confirmed that laughing did strengthen his immune system. He states, "I was greatly elated by the discovery that there is a physiologic basis for the ancient theory that laughter is good medicine." No one, including Cousins himself, would argue that laughter saved him; but it didn't hurt either. It relieved some of his pain and helped him sleep better.

There are many more anecdotal stories of the positive influence of laughter. Many of the concentration camp survivors said that laughing and a sense of humor kept them going, enabling them to survive during those horribly difficult times. Another example is that for many years the popular magazine *Reader's Digest* told funny anecdotal tales under the banner of "Laughter is the Best Medicine." In the same vein, throughout the years, comedians have been the hosts of late night TV shows. People like to conclude their stressful day with laughter.

Please don't laugh (although you can if you like) when I tell you that there are laughing groups that people attend for the sole purpose of enjoying the benefits of laughing. There are also laughing yoga classes for the same purpose. Humorously enough, according to Madeline Vann, a writer on women's health, the first Sunday in May is World Laughter Day. I encourage you to laugh every day, but even more on that one. If you are interested in learning more about the benefits of laughter, check out *Laughter Therapy* by Dr. Goodheart,[17] *Laughter: A Scientific Investigation* by Robert Provine,[18] and *The Healing Power of Humor* by Allen Klein,[19] to name just a few books on this subject.

Klein's book begins with his wife in the hospital with a terminal illness. She playfully hung a male nude centerfold from *Playgirl* above her bed and covered his privates with a plant leaf. As the leaf began to shrivel, they laughed about it. He says:

> Now, Ellen's long illness was hardly a fun time; there were many tense and tearful moments, but there were also periods of laughter. Frequently she would poke me in the ribs and admonish, 'Hey, stop being so morose. I'm still here. We can still laugh together.'

That story reflects why, precisely why, I have included this chapter in my book. Laughing can help you and your loved one in beneficial ways. It can serve to make your experience in Cancerville just a little bit lighter.

Physical Benefits of Laughter

I can't promise that laughing your way through Cancerville will heal or even help all that ails you or your loved one. I won't tell you that it will be good for your head, heart, mind, or soul. I resist the temptation to say it can be a powerful force with preventive and curative value. You must admit that I did sneak it all in though. All of the above may be true or may apply only in certain situations or just for certain people.

What laughter definitely can do is help you release, vent, relax, and dump some of the cess and upset feelings you carry with you in Cancerville. It is a physical and emotional release of energy. Susan made this important point:

> There are also physiological benefits to laughter. It increases oxygenation to the cells and releases those good old endorphins. Also, the activities involved in laughing such as watching a funny movie or show, reading jokes, and the like, help distract us from the pain and the angst, even for a brief time.

Some research studies on laughter suggest that it may be a gentle form of aerobic exercise. Robert Provine, whose book was previously mentioned, is a neuroscientist and laughter researcher. He describes work done by William Fry, who found that it took ten minutes of rowing on his home exercise machine to reach the very same heart rate produced by one minute of hearty laughing. Provine states, "Laughter is the kind of powerful, body-wide act that really shakes up our physiology, a fact that has motivated speculations about its medicinal and exercise benefits since antiquity."

These observations help explain why medical research has found that laughter can actually reduce stress hormones such as cortisol, dopamine, and adrenaline. These hormones are released when we are frightened, worried, or upset. Cancerville certainly promotes high levels of these, and hearty laughter can lower them.

Laughter also increases endorphins and other relaxing and pain-reducing neurotransmitters. In addition, a recent study showed that laughter lowers blood pressure as significantly as when people seriously reduce their salt intake. These findings are no joke. Taken together, they clearly reflect the positive influence laughter can have on our bodies.

In addition, laughter is a nonverbal statement that speaks to the lighter side of life. In its simplest form, it counterbalances the heavies or at least reduces them just a bit. The funny part about laughter is that you don't have to be happy to engage in it. You just need to be willing to see the humor in life events and experiences, despite your unhappiness and worry.

Please don't misinterpret my message. I don't expect you to be happy while your loved one is in Cancerville. I am, however, encouraging you and your loved one to laugh there every once in a while. In truth, you just need to be willing to expose yourself to funny situations. Laughing is usually an involuntary response that occurs automatically. It is both a personal and natural response to whatever tickles your fancy.

Every so often, even in Cancerville, the opportunity presents itself for a humorous comment. It doesn't have to be a major joke—just a giggle or chuckle will do. Recuperating from surgery on a summer day at Sloan-Kettering, Jodi was mobile enough for us all to go to the roof garden to get some fresh air. I immediately noticed all the sad, gray, drained faces sitting and standing all around. I also noticed the elaborate, extra-high fencing. My quip was, "I can't imagine why they feel it necessary to fence in the roof garden." We all chuckled, knowing exactly my meaning. "Darn, we can't jump now," would not have been at all funny. Please, in all instances, know the difference.

In Sum

Some people I help in Cancerville, or with other medical problems, intentionally expose themselves, like Norman Cousins, to comedy. They watch "I Love Lucy" reruns and other funny sitcoms. They listen to funny CDs, go to a comedy club, or watch a cute movie. They tell me that their laughter not only provides an alternative to their tears but also offers a happier vent for their pent-up feelings.

Perhaps laughing and joking have multiple medical and emotional benefits for all. It certainly serves well as a tension release, icebreaker, lightener, and stimulant to our minds and bodies. It generally can reduce people's physical and emotional pain and serve as yet another vent to let go of cess.

In addition, it allows us to get in touch with some of the absurdities of life and Cancerville, as we do our best to dodge their bullets. There is a Jewish saying that translates, "People plan and God laughs." In my humble opinion, we have the right, in and out of Cancerville, to laugh back!

In the next chapter we will talk about communicating in Cancerville. It is a place where words and communication can quickly become as tangled and knotted as a fishing line on a windy day. My goal is to help you prevent such tangles and wrangles from draining your energy.

CHAPTER 20

I will communicate kindly and sensitively.

Communication in Canceerville

Of all the people-related problems in life, communication is certainly the most common. In fact, most problems faced by couples, families, friends, co-workers, and even strangers involve communication breakdowns and failures.

What I observe, both in and out of my office, is that people become defensive and blind to their contributions to communication breakdowns. This can cause even the simplest of topics to turn into heated disagreements and conflicts. The purpose of this chapter is to help you limit, if not avoid, wasting time and energy on these communication snafus.

In Cancerville, communication needs to be clear and sensitive at all times. It is better for all involved when it comes from a cooperative and supportive mindset. In all instances, your goal is to avoid harsh words, needless tension, and conflicts. Speaking through a filter of loving-kindness and seeking a common ground of understanding can make all the difference.

Stress and Cess Can Make a Mess

Despite these goals, communication in any emotionally charged area, especially in Cancerville, can quickly deteriorate in destructive ways. With stress and cess flowing forcefully in Cancerville, communication can easily come undone. Under these pressures and upsets, communication can quickly go off-track like a model train going at too high a speed. Fighting in one war zone is more than enough for you and your loved one to handle. Let's work together to prevent creating any other combative areas.

I fully understand that it is not always easy to leave squabbles and bickering out of Cancerville. Despite our many years together, our love for each other, and our general compatibility, Ronnie and I had our fair share of hot spots. She talked too much in my eyes, I too little in hers. She needed to discuss all of her fears, while I needed not to go there. Her superstitions grated against my attempt to keep my mind rational. My unwillingness to support them made her angry. In my view, a grown man should not have to bite his tongue. Then again, in retrospect, that is so much simpler than fighting about it.

Fortunately, we were able to work through those difficulties and keep moving forward with our eyes on the goal of helping our daughter. To address and reduce our conflicts, I ultimately sought counseling. I needed a female therapist from Venus to help me not be such a Martian.

The purpose of this chapter is to try to help you avoid the traps that distort communication. By doing that, you can prevent the upheaval that can result from hurtful ways of communicating. Both emotionally and practically, your team needs to be strong and united in order to support your loved one. Appropriate communication will contribute to that kind of healthy functioning and enhance everyone's ability to be there for each other.

A Tower of Babel

Though we may all speak the same language, the interpretation of words can often seem like an inkblot test. Everyone perceives and interprets things differently. The "telephone" exercise used in Communication 101 classes demonstrates the distortions that can occur, even in simple interactions. The teacher gives a message to the first student in line and asks that it be whispered to the next student and so on. By the time it gets passed along by six or more students, the message has usually changed in many ways. Sometimes, the last summary sounds nothing like the first. It is both a humorous and telling exercise that shows how easily the heard message can be distorted. When this occurs in real life, feelings can be hurt and sparks may fly.

Many forces combine to cause communication misunderstandings and conflicts. First, we may know what we mean, but that doesn't ensure that we say it in a way that others will clearly understand. I wonder how many times a day someone says to another person, "Oh, I thought you meant..."

A second issue is that we tend to process words differently. In this case we may say what we mean clearly, but the other person misunderstands the message. Yet another miscue is not caused by the words themselves but by the tone in which the words are delivered. If the person's tone sounds critical, sarcastic, upset, etc., it will influence the interpretation of the words themselves. The same is true of facial expressions and body language. Sometimes they are inconsistent with the message, which then lacks credibility and is confusing.

In addition, convenient communication tools like emails and texts can easily ignite sparks of conflict. Because they lack body language, facial expressions, intonation, and other observable cues, they are easy to misinterpret. Compounding the lack of cues is that, at times, we press send prematurely without ensuring that we have expressed ourselves in a kind, understanding, and caring way. In those instances, communication can ping-pong back and forth, causing upset and upheaval to those involved. Yet another problem I have observed and experienced is that it is easier to convey harsh messages when shielded from face-to-face or even phone interaction.

One of the surest ways to create tension and angst is to talk or write to another adult in the tone of a parent-to-child command or criticism. This guarantees that cess will be flowing fast and furiously. We may love our parents, but we didn't always love many times when they were being our parents. I said that in Speech 101 in 1963, and Professor Bednar said, "Penzer, there is hope for you yet!" I'd like to believe he was both perceptive and correct.

Our past experiences, and our cess in particular, affect both how we deliver communication directed toward others and those that are directed toward us. Let's not forget that all of our encounters with others (e.g., a history with an angry father, bossy older sister, unreliable ex-spouse, etc.) are stored in our cesspools and that area occupies quite a large space. All of this can become magnified under the stressful and agitating conditions of Cancerville.

Adult-to-Adult Communication

Authoritative communication, where one person has more clout and power than the other, may work in some organizations such as the military, but it doesn't usually work or sit well in terms of family and friends. This is precisely why people generally, and especially in Cancerville, need to stay in their adult voice and communicate clearly from that position. This is true in Cancerville whether you are talking to the medical team, your loved one, or others. When you speak to others kindly, it is usually reciprocated—perhaps not always, but often enough.

The ultimate in communication breakdown comes in the form of an argument. Once that starts, the communication often deteriorates to child-like levels. Very quickly, the "adults" leave the scene and are replaced by their "junior" counterparts. Hurtful comments and insults can pile one on top of another. Nothing gets resolved, and both parties come away feeling hurt, angry, and unhappy.

In Cancerville, your goal is to stay in your adult position so as not to distract or drain yourself needlessly. Your energies need to be channeled into fighting the cancer enemy, rather than fighting other people. Try to catch yourself when losing control of your communication and move quickly back to adult-to-adult interaction. Should someone else bait you into such a downhill slide, try your best not to bite that sharp hook. Even bickering over simple things (e.g., what time to leave for the doctor appointment, who should pick up the prescription, who will call your loved one, etc.) can trigger needless battles. Your goal is to work cooperatively as a team in all areas of Cancerville.

Please Don't Hurt the Ones You Love

It is ironic that we are often more able to remain adult in our communications with strangers or relatively unimportant people than with our most important family and close friends. Most of us are polite, respectful, and considerate of people we hardly know. Women often complain that their husbands are kind and supportive to a secretary, customer, or co-worker, and yet so blunt and insensitive to them. By the same token, some men have this same complaint about their wives.

I will admit that there have been times when Ronnie requested a discussion "session" with me in my office to get past communication blocks or miscues. The obvious message was that I was kinder, more understanding, and a better communicator at work than at home after a long day of talking to others. Her request woke me up to my need for an attitude adjustment, as it was less expensive than paying my fee!

As the song goes, we often, unintentionally, hurt the ones we love. We don't do this consciously, but somehow learned that we can get away with it. People who love us often forgive us, but I don't encourage you to push your luck; sometimes it can catch up with us. Over time, repeated frustrations and hurts can cause our closest allies to become our enemies. This is why the divorce rate hovers at fifty percent and why family members and good friends stop talking to each other for long periods of time, or sometimes forever.

Few things create tension between spouses like having a loved one in Cancerville. This is even more likely in relationships where there have been previous issues and struggles. If communication breaks down, seek help and support from a counselor who specializes in relationships—preferably someone who also has experience helping people dealing with Cancerville. Work hard to get things resolved as quickly as possible. Think about ways to prevent issues from becoming conflicted. Plan ahead to avoid blow-ups. That is exactly what this couple needed to do in order to avoid a brief but very destructive fight:

Wife: What if, God forbid, he dies?

Husband: I've asked you not to say that to me. I don't want to hear that crap. Shut up.

Wife: Don't tell me to shut up. What if he does? Are you just burying your head in the sand like you always do?

Husband: I'll bury my head, but not him. You need to stop your crazy talk.

Wife: I'm not crazy. You are. People die from cancer every day.

Husband: Stop being so damn negative. If you don't stop, I'm walking out the door.

Obviously, this form of communication serves no purpose and hurts both people at a time when they are already hurting. Think about how you might change the dialogue to make the outcome different. We will look at another version soon.

In the above interaction, the issue of the loved one's prognosis is not trivial, but it is unknown. The feeling of despair versus hope flies in the face of just about everything I have encouraged. However, I fully understand that Cancerville is about scary and unknown outcomes. This wife—the mother of the ailing patient—is realistically worried.

On the flipside, her husband is angry with her for expressing her frightened feelings and going with the darker side of her thoughts. She was begging for reassurance, but his words came across as derogatory and demeaning, and he threatened to walk out and abandon her at a difficult time. In my opinion, this man from Mars takes the prize for insensitivity and mental abuse.

Yet they both contributed to this insensitive outburst. He obviously needed to respond very differently. She, knowing her husband's nature and sensitivities from previous talks, needed to discuss her understandable fears with someone else, even though it was perfectly natural for her to want to share her worst fears with her life partner. Unfortunately, that doesn't always work out well, so it is better to avoid obvious triggers.

She bit the bait and responded in kind to his hurtful words. Directing harsh words towards a person one loves is never helpful. The couple went immediately into their child-based voices, rather than staying in their adult selves. I hope they both apologized to each other within five minutes. There are certain times when the best communicators can have a major meltdown. That is when "I'm sorry dear" can be a very helpful salve, along with a hug.

Here is a redo of the not-so-nice communication presented previously, with a few changes that make a huge difference. Hopefully, you can use it as a model for calmer and more caring communication:

Wife: I know you don't want to think about this, but what if he doesn't make it?

Husband: You are right. I don't want to think about that possibility. I am sorry you are thinking that way. Let's try to assume that everything will be okay and that he will be a survivor, just like the many millions who are doing well.

Wife: But you never know.

Husband: Look dear, such speculations are about as helpful as wondering if we will get into a head-on collision on the way to the hospital today. Please let it go. You are bringing me down at a time I need to be strong and hopeful. If you need to talk about this, please find someone who can handle it. You could call a counselor or talk to the social worker at the hospital.

Wife: Okay, I will. Sorry. Thanks for not getting angry. You are right. Let's go to the hospital. Drive carefully!

That is adult-to-adult conversation personified. It took some respectfulness, caring, and self-restraint, but the result was worth it. In this new version of the conversation, the husband short-circuited the discussion without being hurtful or abusive and pointed his wife in a better direction. Her last comment shows that she understood and appreciated his gentle and supportive response.

I understand that it may seem to you as if no one talks like that. So be the first to communicate in that way, though I doubt that you will be. Some people actually do talk that way, as taking this gentler approach is a win/win for all. This more sensitive way of communicating is not only positive for both of you, but also for your loved one, who needs to be your main focus. I am realistically optimistic you will do your level best to be clear, concise, calm, and caring as you communicate with your Cancerville team of support.

Communicating with Your Loved One Who Has Cancer

There may also be tense times and communication issues between you and your loved one. He or she will likely have fears, discouraged feelings, and moody moments, as well as a variety of other emotions. Fatigue and pain wear down a person's dam. All of this and more can make for a less than ideal communication experience.

Let's look at another example of a hurtful scene—this one between a mother and adult daughter with cancer. It is a bit extreme, but an encounter that actually happened. It was a communication breakdown of grand proportion. Ronnie has asked me to reassure you that it wasn't a dialogue between her and Jodi. Personally, I feel you clearly know that already:

Mother: I hate what chemo does to you.

Daughter: Me too. I feel like crap.

Mother: Maybe you shouldn't have any more? It's poison.

Daughter: Mom, we've been through this before. The doctors say it is important.

Mother:	But look what it does to you. It breaks my heart to see you like this.
Daughter:	Then go home. I don't need your negativity on top of what I am already dealing with.
Mother:	I guess I can't do anything right in your eyes. I might as well be dead.
Daughter:	How the hell did this all of a sudden become about you? I hate when you do that.
Mother:	Oh, so now you hate me. That chemo is affecting your mind as well as your body. It kills people, you know.
Daughter:	Thank you very much for that news bulletin. I thought mothers were supposed to help their children.
Mother:	I'm going to kill myself.
Daughter:	Me too (her bedroom door is slammed loudly shut as both begin to cry).

This mother needed to voice her fears and feelings to someone/anyone other than her daughter. It was an outrageously unfair rant made worse by the daughter feeling weak after her round of chemo. The best thing the daughter could have done was to go to her room as soon as the topic came up and say, "Mom, I'm going to lie down now. Thanks for coming over." Even better would be if mom could stop herself from putting her worries on her daughter.

Being patient and understanding, and staying in your adult mindset and voice, will help to limit these cess-based bursts from becoming burning battles. As I have previously said, sometimes the best form of communication is a wordless hug. Other times, you may just cry together and give each other support. Of course, there are times when words can work and when you can, by example, encourage adult-based conversation.

There may be times when your loved one is in a bad mood and lashes out at you in some way. If you feel yourself being drawn into a conflict with your angry, hurting, and/or worn-out loved one, you can say to yourself: "Self, this is what Bill meant. Now is not the time to bite the provocative bait; just respond kindly, caringly, lovingly, and helpfully." Or you can say to your loved one: "I am sorry you are so upset. Is there anything I can do to be helpful? If not, I will let you be for a while." Then, just pause, hug, exit, and return in fifteen to thirty minutes.

Differences Between Men and Women

There is yet another issue with which we all need to reckon. Men and women have different natures. As John Gray taught us years ago, *Men are From Mars, Women are From Venus*.[20] Once we understand this framework, it's not terribly hard to understand why we encounter challenges as we all try to live together on Planet Earth. This is what got Adam and Eve in so much trouble way back when, and it has been strained between men and women ever since.

Dr. Gray has repeatedly said that men and women have different coping strategies, especially under stressful conditions. Men, he has suggested, cope by solving problems; they are frustrated when that is not easy to do. Clearly, men's frustrations in Cancerville are at very high levels. This is one of the many reasons men get very depressed there. Their will and problem solving efforts are thwarted in Cancerville in so many ways. Yet, as we previously saw, there are many things they can do there to be helpful.

In contrast, women, as Gray has pointed out, want to talk about the source of their stress. They just need to vent and seek support and understanding. They often get upset when their man rushes in to try to fix things. Many women have said to me, "I did not ask him for solutions. I just wanted him to listen, understand, and support me. All I needed was a kind word and a hug." We foolish Martians rush in to "fix it" and if that fails, try our hardest to forget it as fast as we can. There are times, in and out of Cancerville, when we Martians just need to be patient listeners, kind-hearted friends, and sources of strength and support.

My hope is that you and your spouse or other team members can have a meeting of the mind. The key is talking it out together in an adult-to-adult manner and finding points of compromise. You can also avoid arguing about trivial issues or having debates about that which is unknown. Try to pay attention to repetitive hurtful themes so you can catch your communication drifting in that direction and intervene preventively.

When things are coming at you quickly in Cancerville, reason and rationality tend to be the first to go. I hope you can blow a whistle, call a time-out, calm yourself, cooperate, and work together with those closest to you. If all else fails, you can learn or relearn the art of apology. Sometimes a simple "sorry dear" is all that it takes to get your communication and comaraderie back on track. And if your partner needs you to knock on wood, bite your tongue, or whatever it takes to ward off the evil spirits, indulge him or her. Who knows, maybe those actually work—poo, poo, poo!

Giving Yourself Permission to Avoid Toxic People

In some instances, the best option is to limit or avoid communicating with some people. Most everyone means well, but not everyone does well. Try to avoid or limit your interactions with people whose influence becomes toxic in a variety of ways. Watch out for the hysterics and the pessimists and especially the ones that combine both. Also, be sure to avoid the narcissists who insist in one way or another that "it" is all about them. Be watchful of those who think they are doctors and know it all or those who believe they can predict the future. All of this can twist your mind into a pretzel of pessimism at a time when you need to try your hardest to stay positive.

You will know you have encountered a toxic person by how you feel when you conclude the conversation; you will feel as if you were a cartoon character just run over by a bulldozer. You will also feel drained, upset, angry, and perhaps even hurt. You will wish the encounter never happened.

If you realize you are with a toxic person, try not to be mean, but do be assertively self-protective. Toxic people add cess to your pool while simultaneously kicking holes in your dam. The strange thing is that they think they have been oh so helpful in which case you need to be oh so unavailable. Encouraging permission for this self-protection is a very important piece of advice.

What should you do if the toxic person is a family member, close friend, or even life partner? You can ask them nicely to be more sensitive to your needs at this difficult time. Calmly discuss your feelings, citing examples of times they added to your upset or were otherwise insensitive. If they cannot change their communication, you will need to find ways to block their toxic intrusions. In a couple of instances, Ronnie and I discontinued communicating with people close to us whose toxicity added to our burden in Cancerville. No one, and I mean no one, has the right to add to your cess and stress—especially not while you and your loved one are dealing with cancer!

The Value of a Support Net

If you find that, despite my suggestions and words of encouragement, your communication is not working well, consider getting feedback from a counselor. As previously discussed in Chapter 17, "Having a Counselor and/or Support Group in Your Corner," sometimes, smart as we may be, we need some feedback and guidance from others. No one has perfect communication skills. That is why Ronnie edits my writings. This happens after I have edited a chapter several times. We work on it again, and often again and again, until it feels right, is clear, and flows well. Then Kerri comes in, like the sweepers at the end of a parade, and cleans up what we missed and left behind.

A counselor is to the mind what an editor is to written communication. In day-to-day interactions, though, no one has the lag time of the writer's luxury. When we talk, we basically shoot from the hip. A counselor can help us learn how to do that better and avoid shooting ourselves in the foot. He or she can help us find the "delete key" in our mind, so we can use it when necessary, and also help us find a more caring voice with which to communicate. Both counselors and editors are word teachers who help refine, refresh, rephrase, and redo our messages. My "editor" wife, Ronnie, my editor, Kerri, and my therapist, Karen, have all been extremely helpful to me.

In Sum

In most conflicts, both parties could have made different choices if they were in their rational, healthy adult mindsets. When you're fatigued, stressed, and overwhelmed in Cancerville, it's hard not to regress to a more combative state. Yet a little awareness and effort to control that can go a long way. Having read this chapter, you can now tune into those moments when you start to move toward negative communication and stop yourself, even in mid-sentence, before the conversation gets too out of control.

People in Cancerville need to speak in a way that fortifies rather than vilifies. I am hopeful that you can find a voice that will communicate your messages accurately and appropriately. I am also hopeful that those around you will do the same. In all of life, and particularly in Cancerville, our healthy adult choices and voices need to prevail. I am confident you agree and will work toward that difficult but doable goal.

Let's now move on to talk about leaving Cancerville behind. This is not always easy to do as it follows us in one way or another. Perhaps the best we can expect is to just put some distance between Cancerville and ourselves.

PART V

Putting Distance Between Yourself and the Land

CHAPTER 21

I will be able to get through this.

No One Really Knows Where the Road Goes

I debated not including most of this chapter because it confronts loss in Cancerville. Ultimately, I decided that, much as I have tried to be positive, hopeful, and inspiring, my philosophy of realistic optimism demands that I be clear and honest. This book would not be complete if I glossed over the harsher side of Cancerville. If all is going well in your Cancerville experience, feel free to skip to the section titled, "Meant to Be: Moving Forward Hopefully," page 210.

Not Meant to Be

At some point there is a wide and sharp fork in the Cancerville road. It can come weeks, months, or even years after the diagnosis. One way continues life while the other concludes it. Hopefully, your loved one is among the fortunate ones in the former group.

Sadly, painfully, and poignantly, some reading this will be among those who lose their loved one in Cancerville. I am sincerely sorry for that. Losing a loved one in or out of Cancerville is an inconsolable experience. There are no words to be said, only prayers and tears; for some there are only tears. It is a mind-boggling, gut-wrenching, and heartbreaking experience.

Trying to Cope with Loss

How do you cope when Cancerville has robbed you of your loved one? How do you accept having followed my encouragement to turn down the spotlight on catastrophe only to have it shine so brightly that it burns your eyes, forcing them to close? How do you accept defeat and such a grievous loss in the war zone of Cancerville? Resentfully. Bitterly. Miserably. Sadly. Slowly. Very slowly! Loss involves all of the above, plus much more, then squared and squared again.

Some never fully accept their inequitable loss. They limp along, going through the motions without ever being able to absorb and let go of their pain-filled emotions. Many others heal sufficiently in due time to pick up the fragile pieces of their lives and move forward. A few people, like Nancy Brinker, go on to accomplish amazing things as a memorial to their loved one. Some find ways to memorialize their loved one in a simpler manner. Their rage and hurt over their loss fuels them to make a difference.

Some people who have lost their loved one seek out counseling support, bereavement groups, and/or books that help heal deep wounds. Others seek out spiritual comfort. There is, no doubt, support on the Internet too. Some just heal in their own way, in their own time, on their own.

Another Family Loss in Cancerville

Cancerville came and smacked us upside the head once again yesterday as Ronnie and I were continuing to make our way through New Zealand. We learned via email on our cruise ship that my first cousin Debra died less than six weeks after being diagnosed. She was a dedicated mother to her adult twin children, Naomi and Alan, as well as a dedicated physician. My cousin was largely responsible for my mom living to one hundred. Debra had been her personal, "still made house calls" doctor for more than twenty years. Ironically, Mom outlived her by sixteen days, never knowing that her niece had passed at age sixty-two.

A common feeling that many have, and one I had momentarily after reading the email, was that all my cousin's treatments these last six weeks were a painful waste of her time and energy. She had major surgery and two other related surgeries, causing her needless suffering. My initial reaction was that it was all for naught. The trouble is that once we know of a loss, we are easily led to that incorrect conclusion.

The truth is that neither the medical team nor you know the outcome before it occurs. No one can predict the future. No one knows how a person's Cancerville story will turn out. In my cousin's case, hindsight tells us that much of what occurred in the name of treatment served no purpose. At the time, however, the surgeries were essential to try and save her life. It would be like stopping CPR prematurely because the person was taking "too long" to respond. There is a sign in my office that reads, "Never, Never, Never Give Up!" My simple belief about fighting any life and death battle is that we should never give up unless and until we have no choice but to accept the very sad reality.

Hope for the Future

Coincidently, on the last day of our cruise, we learned that Holland America Line sponsors an "On Deck for the Cure" 5K walk and donates the proceeds to Susan G. Komen organization. We learned that in the past few years Holland America has presented the foundation with over two million dollars. They have this walk on every one of their ships on every cruise. Well done and bravo! Nancy Brinker has been a master at having major corporations join her fundraising efforts.

Each participant, after making a donation, received a tee shirt, a pink rubber bracelet, and an opportunity to walk ten times around the deck in a "race" for the cure. This was a formidable challenge after eating and drinking for a couple of weeks on the cruise. Both Ronnie and I joined in and completed all ten laps around the ship. We were one of the last to finish, just before a couple of eighty-year-olds, but that we finished was what was important to us.

Though this experience did not lessen the pain of losing my cousin prematurely, it did rekindle the flame of our hopes for the future. It made us think about those whose burdens will be eased because of people's generous contributions, new protocols and their targeted delivery, more efficient and effective treatments, and leaps of knowledge forward. We went from loss and deep sadness back to hope filled with love. This powerful emotional experience, coming just at the time we needed it, helped start the healing process that will allow us over time to accept our most recent loss in Cancerville.

The Five Stages of Grief

I had much respect for Dr. Elizabeth Kubler-Ross' work and book, *On Death and Dying* when I read it in the early 1970's.[21] I was, however, never comfortable with or convinced of the idea that people went through different stages as they mourned and grieved their loss.

She believed that the stages were denial, anger, bargaining, depression, and eventually acceptance. Though the interpretation was that this sequence applied to grieving a loved one, she was, interestingly enough, actually writing about the stages we go through to accept our own death potentials.

I have always viewed people as being more dynamic and fluid in their mindly matters and never agreed with the idea of an orderly sequence of stages. I have seen and experienced the grieving process to be more of a back and forth flow of emotions until one can slowly move on.

Such fluidity of feelings is consistent with the cesspool and dam model that is based on the ebb and flow of thoughts and emotions. In all emotional healing, no matter the issue, I have never observed a straight line of consistently forward progress. Nor have I seen a simple sequence of stages through which people pass. In my observation and experience, the resolution of emotional issues is never that orderly.

Ruth Davis Koningsberg's book, *The Truth About Grief,*[22] presents evidence to contradict the idea of staged grieving. Research done by Yale University found that acceptance of the loved one being gone was present from the very beginning of the grief process. The people interviewed yearned for their loved one as opposed to feeling anger or depression. The book quotes psychologist Janice Genevro as saying:

> The information being used to help the bereaved was misaligned with the latest research, which increasingly indicates that grief is not a series of steps that ultimately deposit us at a psychological finish line, but rather a grab bag of symptoms that come and go and, eventually, simply lift.

Clearly, these results confirm my observations and allow for a wide range of emotions to be part of your mourning process. There is no "right" way to experience your grief. Your hurt, angry, depressed, sad, and other feelings will flow randomly for quite a while. Hopefully, you will find sources of comfort and support as you heal from your loss.

Do What Works Best for You

People vary widely in their nature and their needs. One person's meat is truly another's poison. There are many paths to emotional healing and I am confident that you will choose those that are most suited to you.

For some people, counseling and/or a support group are seen as helpful. They find comfort in the support and encouragement, and they like having a sounding board and a place to cry without feeling self-conscious. Others do not feel comfortable with these supports and find different ways to vent their feelings. Still others will not vent and just stoically move forward.

Practically speaking, I believe that most people know themselves well enough to determine what they need and what will work for them. I encourage you to avoid or at least discount people who preach a rigid system that says, "You must work through your grief and loss and heal from it or you will never be okay," or, "Unless you do your grief work, your mourning will be incomplete." I believe there are many paths to accepting and resolving painful realities—you need to find the one(s) that fit and work best for you.

I think my mom is a perfect example of this very idea. Having kept her faculties and mobility for almost ninety-nine years, she grieved repeatedly. Many young family members and just about all of her contemporaries, many of whom were much younger than she, passed away. Yet to my knowledge, she never sought counseling for that or any other issues. Mom went to the gym regularly until she was over ninety-eight years old, was fiercely independent, and actively participated in community and reading study groups, all while having a core friend group of mostly younger women.

In addition, she laughed and cried often and with each death seemed to strengthen her resolve to live a healthy, balanced life. She did the latter better than anyone I know; she took charge of every aspect of her life with a positive, can-do spirit. At ninety-seven she planned her own funeral and was adamant about being buried in a traditional plain pine box with a brief graveside service. That I gave the eulogy tells you it was hardly brief.

Prior to her dementia and eventual passing, my mother, a wise and learned woman, was reading Ernest Becker's brilliant Pulitzer Prize winning book, *The Denial* of Death.[23] She was obviously trying to get out of denial and into accepting the inevitability of her own passing. She did life and death her way, and I encourage you, in this spirit, to do the same in struggling to accept your loss and move slowly forward. Mom's unique life is summarized on her memorial website at www.sadiethelady.me.

Making Peace with Your Loss

Tony told me that his mother went through three difficult years after being diagnosed with ovarian cancer. She had intermittent chemo throughout and ultimately died of a heart attack. Though she passed at sixty-five, he said he was at peace when she died.

In those three years, he spent much time with her and was always there for her when she needed him. They were very close in the last few weeks, even though he did not know she was going to pass. She was initially given a fifteen percent chance of living one to three years. That she beat the odds helped her family and Tony accept her fate and begin to heal. As I have said, in life, and particularly in Cancerville, everything is relative. We need to appreciate the time we have had, as much as feel sad for the time we lost.

Just the other day, I received a condolence card from the hospice that took care of my mother. Inside the card was another called "The Mourner's Bill of Rights." I had never seen it before, but want to share it with you now because it might just be of help.

You have the right to:

- experience your own unique grief
- talk about your grief
- feel a multitude of emotions

- be tolerant of your physical and emotional limits
- experience "griefbursts"
- make use of ritual
- embrace your spirituality
- search for meaning
- treasure your memories
- move toward your grief and heal

As a mourner you have many rights. Exercising them will help you grieve and move forward. We are all here on borrowed time, and we never get to know in advance when our time is going to be up.

It was Shakespeare who reminded us that our candles are brief and will eventually go out. As I recently told my friend Eileen, "I need to finish this book. Though healthy, I feel like I am in a footrace with destiny." In truth, every day, in every way, we all are. As if to add an exclamation point to the last sentence, Eileen was diagnosed with cancer less than a month after I made that statement. She entered Cancerville strongly and with a positive attitude and is doing very well.

Bernie Siegel, M.D., said it best in *Love, Medicine and Miracles*: "No one lives forever; therefore, death is not the issue. Life is. Death is not a failure. Not choosing to take on the challenge of life is." Throughout this book I have encouraged you to take on the challenges of Cancerville. At the end of the day, that is really all we can do.

Meant to Be—Moving Forward Hopefully

Those for whom the fork in the Cancerville road turns toward life are very, very fortunate indeed, but unfortunately still do not have an easy time. It is, undeniably, a long and winding road with many hairpin turns, speed bumps, and detours. Being a survivor is a Pyrrhic victory. If you Google that or search for it in your old-fashioned Webster's, you will find that a Pyrrhic victory refers to a battle won despite many significant costs and losses.

No one leaves Cancerville unscathed by the experience. We are all wounded warriors on its battlefield.

There is never certainty in Cancerville, no matter how long ago the initial diagnosis was made. Just ask any survivor, parent, or partner how he or she feels a day or two before the patient goes for an annual, semiannual, or quarterly checkup. It is a worrisome, anxiously anticipatory time analogous to a jury returning to the courtroom for a critical verdict. In Cancerville, there are no double-jeopardy rules. You are all on trial each time for the crime cancer has perpetrated on your loved one. Your loved one goes to the hospital for X-rays, MRIs, blood work, scans, etc., and you go to the bathroom for a case of the runs.

This is the realistic part of realistic optimism. Though I continue to encourage you to take an "all will be well" position, I fully understand that checkups may not be comfortable times for your loved one or for you. Each test becomes a measure of hope potentials. That critical day is a "too high staked poker game" for most of us. Having been already worn down by Cancerville, and having learned enough to know that cancer can reoccur, those test days become a foot-tapping, finger-rapping, mind-trapping time. Hopefully, the tools we previously discussed will calm and support you through these stressful times.

It is my sincere hope that those times pass quickly for you and the results continue to be favorable. May the verdict be a reprieve for your loved one, so that he or she can go on and continue to enjoy his or her life. Assume that will be the case with every checkup.

You Really Never Leave Cancerville Behind

These uneasy times and the nature of the territory are why you don't ever really leave Cancerville. You and your loved one can put distance between yourselves and Cancerville, but it follows along like slow-moving gray clouds overhead no matter how many years have passed. What were once minor problems, such as your loved one having a headache, stomach upset, rash, fatigue, or bloody nose, can all take on more worrisome dimensions for the family as well as for the survivor. When these are confirmed to be what they appear, and not signs of anything more serious, your mind can return to a calmer place.

In addition, every time you hear about a famous person or anyone else being diagnosed with or passing from cancer, your own personal Cancerville experience will flit through your mind like a black cat in a dark alley. Imagine what Elizabeth Edwards losing her long, strongly fought battle did to survivors and their families. Cancerville stories of the rich and famous, as well as the not-so-well-known, appear to be rising like the price of gas.

Then again, we can each choose to focus on positive outcomes. Former First Lady Betty Ford passed from natural causes at the age of 93. She was diagnosed with breast cancer in 1974, a time when the word "breast" was hardly spoken in public, especially by someone in a prominent position. She was a courageous and outspoken "balls to the walls" woman who openly declared her disease. She later dealt directly with her addiction and subsequently opened the Betty Ford Center to help others with drug and alcohol related problems. She was truly a first lady who made a difference. Clearly, we can choose to focus on the fact that she was treated for cancer at a time when little was known and managed to live thirty-seven years post-diagnosis.

It is, however, likely that relevant news, magazine articles, or TV programs will now take on a special significance for you. Cancer breakthroughs will be silently applauded, while sad news will likely hit you in a sensitive spot. As Ronnie and I did the 5K walk on the ship, we felt very differently about the experience from those who were just being Good Samaritans. We were survivors by proxy and, if we had to, would have finished that walk on our knees.

In addition, October, which is Breast Cancer Awareness Month, is not an easy one for us. We are aware—much too aware! All of the media focus brings it all back for millions of people as well as for us. Though we support pink in every way, we can't deny our feelings that it all really, really stinks! Here again, feel free to insert the word before stinks that Ronnie doesn't allow me to include.

Fortunately, as time goes by, your Cancerville-related thoughts will lessen, and slowly, but surely, life will return to greater and greater normalcy for all concerned. Will you still think about it from time to time? Absolutely. Will it dominate your waking moments to the extent it once did? Not likely. As some say, it is a "new normal" which will take you some time to adjust to. All things considered, despite it being a Pyrrhic victory, I am confident that you appreciate and feel grateful for your loved one's survival.

As a result of that appreciation, many in this group set their sights on helping those still in or who will be coming into Cancerville. They may volunteer at a hospital, donate money, organize or participate in fundraisers, and do special things for the good of the cause. Our son Mike grew his hair long so he could donate it to Wigs for Kids.

In addition, he recently lived his dream and played in the main event of the World Series of Poker in Las Vegas, Nevada. Though he didn't come in the money, he did come in better than seventy-five percent of the almost seven thousand player field. He recently told us that while there he signed up to donate one percent of his winnings to a poker-related fundraiser for cancer. Maybe next time! He did win a much smaller tournament while there and happily sent in their share. Rob's fundraiser in November is another example, and knowing him, he will aim higher than the sixty thousand dollars they collected last year. I will update you on a future Cancerville.com Facebook post.

In Sum

All of the above is undeniable, as are the blessings when your loved one becomes a survivor. Though those who have entered Cancerville are never quite the same, winning any battle in these trenches is huge. It is David finally slaying the mighty Goliath with his small but powerful slingshot.

Despite its hardships, Cancerville does teach many life lessons. Let us turn our attention to them as we continue to heal and begin to slowly conclude our journey together. We have come a long way walking side-by-side, and by now I am hopeful my words have helped you in many ways.

CHAPTER 22

I will focus on what I learned in Cancerville.

Helpful Life Lessons You Can Learn from Your Cancerville Experience

Life teaches us lessons in many ways and from many different places. Beyond formal education, much is learned from the streets of our life's journey. It is important that we pay attention and take in new information wherever we go. Such is the case in Cancerville. Much as we hate being there, we can learn a great deal from this experience. That its streets are dark, scary, and mean doesn't mean that we can't learn from them.

Even though we are worn, weary, and wounded from Cancerville, we can still come away with some heightened awareness and new perspectives. Lance Armstrong concludes his previously referenced book by saying, "Cancer no longer consumes my life, my thoughts, or my behavior, but the changes it wrought are there in me, unalterable."

We have spent enough time on the painful lessons we learn in Cancerville and how to combat all that negativity. I hope that some of my words have helped you to salve that pain and come at your experience from a different angle. I would like for us to begin to wind down our journey by looking at the more positive lessons you may have learned—ones that I know I did. Most if not all of the positive lessons were not new bits of information as much as pearls of wisdom that can easily get lost in the hustle-bustle of everyday life.

Gratitude Helps Your Attitude

Strange as it may sound, I feel grateful for rediscovering gratitude while in Cancerville. Of all I took away, this stands out as very significant. Gratitude nourishes our attitude and many other feelings. I have come to believe that gratitude is milk for our minds. Got gratitude? I can't quite figure out what to smear above my upper lip, or how to do that because I have a moustache, but that isn't important.

Too often in our quest for more, we forget to acknowledge and appreciate what we already have. I am not only talking about appreciating our food, clothing, and shelter, given that many around the world lack those very basics. I am also referring to having our physical and emotional health, support from loved ones, opportunities to stretch and grow, goals that have been achieved and are in process, and occasional times that are fun, happy, and warm.

I am also talking about waking up in the morning and having something worthwhile to occupy our time, having our faculties and mobility, and even enjoying simple things such as a pleasant meal with a special person. In a spiritually oriented book, *Turn My Mourning into Dancing*,[24] Henri Nouwen quotes a friend who, upon moving away, said:

> We are thankful for all the good things that have happened, for all the friendships we have developed, for all the hopes that have been realized. We simply have to try to accept the painful moments.

The reason Cancerville reminded me to get back to gratitude was how ungrateful I felt about being there. From the vantage point of Cancerville, I could look back on everything I had in my life before that time and appreciate it in a whole new way. I took much too much for granted before we entered Cancerville, and I didn't want to keep doing that. With this new perspective, my gratitude bank, like my pride bank, now runs over with thanks for the most basic blessings in my life. I hope the same is true for you.

I also realize that it may take a while for those still enmeshed in Cancerville to feel comfortable or grateful. I understand how easy it is in Cancerville to feel that you have nothing for which to be thankful. Try to use the wide-angle lens we discussed in Chapter 16 to take in more than the difficult Cancerville scene. From that view, it is likely you will find some things for which to feel grateful, despite your present situation. If you can do that, it will help offset some of the painful times through which you are now living. I speak from experience when I repeat that gratitude is milk for your mind. Get gratitude and don't worry about your upper lip—just keep it stiff for the moment.

Everything is Truly Relative

If you go back to the first chapter of this book, you can see the scale that shows my "theory of relativity." An important life lesson that Cancerville teaches us is to be better able to see the difference between that which is truly important and that which is relatively not. All of a sudden, Cancerville provides a new yardstick by which to measure life and what happens to us. I am hopeful that you will no longer exaggerate the more minor issues that you face if, in fact, you are prone to doing that.

After Cancerville, it is not easy to go back to the magnifying glasses in your mind that enlarge the less important problems that come along. Whatever measuring instruments we carry inside our heads have the potential to automatically adjust and recalibrate as a result of having been to Cancerville.

A clear example occurred during one of our visits to New York for one of Jodi's chemo treatments. While we were there, Hurricane Wilma visited our neighborhood and home in South Florida. When it rains it pours, especially during a hurricane—and most especially in Cancerville. Flights were cancelled, and we stayed in New York for a few extra days, which gave us more time with Jodi and Zev.

We asked our friends Esther and Alex to drive by our house and report back to us. The downed trees and lack of working traffic lights convinced Alex that such an undertaking was too dangerous—so Esther went alone. Had we been more aware of the conditions we would not have asked her to go. Fortunately, she made it safely to our home and back to hers. She reported that our home had taken a major hit. Our swimming pool had morphed into an overflowing cesspool filled with trees, leaves, assorted debris, and even a patio chair—better our swimming pool than our minds!

To give you a sense of the extensive damage, we paid $11,000 just to have the downed trees in our backyard cut up, removed from our roof, pool deck, and pool, and moved to the front yard. The other estimate was $18,000. Believe me when I say that the homes in our neighborhood are not mansions and the lots are pretty small.

How much did the hurricane damage upset us? Not one bit! Even Ronnie, who tends to get more upset about those kinds of things than I do, took it in stride. It was all just stuff that could be repaired or replaced.

I could finally fully embrace a sign that has been on a shelf in our library for many years. The sign says: "Les choses importantes de la vie ne sont pas des choses." That translates to: "The important things in life are not things." This statement is undeniably true in all ways, but it feels especially true after one has been to Cancerville.

Cancerville helped us both realize that the damage to our home was not significant compared to the damage to our daughter and ourselves. Few things in life are actually more serious or significant than cancer; that lesson is learned the day you arrive in Cancerville. Actually, even before that day, I used to say to myself: "If it ain't chemo, it ain't nothin'!" as a way to keep whatever issue I was facing in my life relative and in perspective. I understand that my English teachers would not have been impressed.

Priority of the Minority

Just as your yardstick shifts after being in Cancerville, so do your priorities. What once was so important comes down a peg or two or more. Similarly, what may have once been unimportant now takes on much more significance. Working hard, earning a living, and setting and achieving goals are still important, but people often have an epiphany after being in Cancerville. That experience expands our awareness of the dangers that lurk about and of the importance of taking better care of ourselves. Time in Cancerville can easily push us to find balance and to strive to hold that course. This experience leans heavily on us to prioritize setting healthy goals and sticking to them. It helps us appreciate each day and use it to our advantage. While work is important, other priorities are added to our personal equation.

Of course, there are no guarantees that taking better care of you will always make a difference. There are many well-known examples of people who were very fit, yet took a major health hit. Not too many people were as fit as Lance Armstrong, multi-winner of the Tour de France, was when he was diagnosed with metastasized testicular cancer at age twenty-five. Two-time Olympic gold medal winning gymnast, Shannon Miller, was also fit when she was diagnosed with a form of ovarian cancer at age thirty-three.

Similarly, Jodi was the healthiest member of our family; her diet and exercise regimen were solid. At the time she entered Cancerville, she was a gyrotonic personal fitness trainer who taught others to use that interesting technology to work out. Go figure! What we try to do to help ourselves be healthier doesn't always work, but hopefully it does increase our odds.

As we know, life offers no guarantees. But Darwin did get it right—the odds generally favor the survival of the fittest. Lance, Shannon, and Jodi's in-shape fitness did not prevent or protect them from Cancerville, but perhaps it did help them become survivors. Similarly, perhaps you will commit to being fitter just as I am trying to do. I will fit into that suit from six years ago—one of these days. Of that I am certain, well almost certain. As we have learned, in life nothing is for sure.

A Stitch in Time Allows for a Switch in Lifestyle

One of the many shifts people often experience after having been to Cancerville is how they allocate their time. All of a sudden, as part of the changes in perspective and priority, time is made for many things that may have previously been given less importance. This includes fitting in family visits, fun times, that elusive though relaxing yoga class, or whatever else is on your "taking care of self" list.

As an observer of people, I have come to realize that many of us are self-sacrificing to a fault. We cater to others, our jobs, community, church or temple, and to a host of causes other than ourselves. Somewhere in the maze of life we get lost. There is not enough time to go around, and our piece of the proverbial pie gets smaller and smaller.

Oftentimes, we just get some occasional crumbs, and that is a crummy way to live. It assumes that we will go on forever and ever and eventually play catch-up. It is based on the belief that eventually we will take that class or whatever it is that we have no time to do now. As Cancerville reminds us, there is no catch-up in life; there is only now. So *carpe diem*! No one's future, in or out of Cancerville, is for sure.

Though in theory it should not take a trip to Cancerville to cure the problem of not allotting more time for you, your having been there can be a mighty motivator. As a result of your experience there, you realize that your time is not infinite. You come to know that no alarm will be sounded to warn you of an impending problem or to give you time to squeeze in what's important to you just before the crisis hits.

Hopefully, you have come to realize that you have worth, are special, and deserve a fairer slice of that tasty, glop-free pie. I sincerely hope that you will come away from your Cancerville experience with a sense of entitlement to more than you might have allowed yourself in the past. In my opinion, you have earned the right to calmer experiences and will hopefully choose to steer some of your time in that direction. At the very least, I hope you will draw upon the relaxing, natural tools for healing that I have encouraged.

Strengthening of Character

As we headed into Cancerville, I told Jodi that she would become an even stronger person by having to deal with all of the challenges. Did she believe me at the time? Was this statement even encouraging to her in the midst of all that was going on? Maybe she believed me or maybe not. But I truly believed that prediction at the time and still feel that it was true.

We all came out stronger from this experience. We learned that we could take on Cancerville and make the land our own in the same ways I have encouraged you to do. We learned how to stare it down and take charge. We found that little got in our way or blocked our path. If it did, we knocked it over—if not with a flick of our wrists, with a kick to its groin. We were, in fact, "balls to the walls," and rose to the challenges like strong athletes. My friend Rob also showed his character and strength in his journey in all the many things he was able to accomplish for his family and for Cancerville. He, like Jodi, is an even stronger person today. Of that I am certain.

Like Rob was for his family, Jodi was our team captain, just as she was for her Taravella High School drill team. She helped us keep marching strongly and gracefully along as she led the way. Nothing was too much for her or, as a result, for us. There was no stretch that she or we couldn't handle.

Our game plan was definitely in effect as we slowly adapted to a new world order of disorder. I grew stronger as we went along although chemo days were always rough around the edges for me. Just like Jodi, we silently and stoically accepted what came her way. We looked Goliath in the face, and every single time we needed to, we whipped out our slingshots and hit him squarely between the eyes. "Take that you…!" Ronnie is one tough editor.

Ties that Bind and are Kind

Cancerville fosters closeness in all directions. As your support team forms and grows, I hope you will all work together for the good of your loved one's cause. Over time, winning teams develop winning ways and closer feelings. Family members and friends, some who have not been close in the past, come to the fore like a racehorse on steroids. It is not only the time spent together that forges these ties, but also the combined energy spent climbing challenging Cancerville mountains.

Jodi and Zev are closer with each other and with us as well. Ronnie and I are as close as we have ever been, fostered by our Cancerville experience as well as her editing this book with me. In fact, our whole family seems to be closer since our Cancerville experience. Positive, cooperative energies flow even more now, and family gatherings take on a special meaning. These gatherings now include the adult twin children of my cousin Debra.

Remember way back when I said I didn't really know Rob and that he was my friend's son? Rob and I are now buddies for life, united by Cancerville's common cause. We are two fathers who have walked the mean streets of Cancerville together, like those tough cops I mentioned in a crime-infested neighborhood.

We kicked some butt together and didn't allow ours to get too bruised! He just invited us to come to Rye, New York and participate in this year's fundraising walk in November. Jake will be leading it carrying a white balloon as a survivor, and Chase will carry a red one as his key supporter. We will be there in a happy heartbeat.

Trauma seems to bind people to one another as much as happy times do. Perhaps it is as simple as wanting to savor every moment of togetherness, having come to realize that it is far from guaranteed. I hope you too will experience this unique form of bonding with your family and friends. It is also why I said early on that while you and I may never meet face-to-face, there might be a special chemistry that forms between us. I hope it has been that way for you.

In Sum

There are probably many more positive life lessons to be learned from your Cancerville experience than those I have described here. In fact, I am sure you will discover more along the way. I have certainly worked less and played more in the past six years: "If not now, when?" I asked myself.

Some people, after their Cancerville experience, decide to volunteer in some way. I increased that part of my life as well. Such good deeds often come back to reward you in many ways, not the least of which are pride bank deposits. In the final analysis, those are even better than piggy bank ones. Research consistently shows that people who do good deeds and help others feel happier. There may be some other positive lessons, too, which will be unique to you. Feel free to share them with me at bill@cancerville.com.

I am finally eager and excited to share the amazing fairy tale experience Jodi, Zev, Ronnie, and I had and enjoyed so much as we gratefully but cautiously distanced ourselves from Cancerville. This tale is forever tattooed in my brain just like July 8, 2005. But it is a much more beautiful image—it has love written all over it!

Never in our wildest imaginations could we have anticipated in 2005 that in 2009 we would be… Please keep reading to find out how we went from the outhouse of Cancerville to the penthouse of life. Our story shows that we just never know what the future has in store for any of us. I am sure you will find our fairy tale uplifting and inspirational, which is one reason I saved it for the conclusion of our walk together.

CHAPTER 23

I hope for happier, calmer, and better times.

A Modern Day Fairy Tale

I want to finally share the magical fairy tale dream trip we took a few years after my family's nightmarish times in Cancerville. I assure you that it is completely true without embellishment or exaggeration.

In 2008, we were finally feeling a little better. Although Jodi was still taking Tamoxifen, she was past the heavy-duty chemo and, though a bit tired, feeling much better. As I had previously assured myself, her hair had grown back. Her relationship with her partner, Zev, was very positive. They were starting to enjoy life again, and so were Ronnie and I.

A Seed is Planted

Our son Michael called around that time and told us he was going to an annual breast cancer fundraiser within his industry. He described a trip they were auctioning for four people. Much as he would have liked to go with us, he thought it would be more fitting for us to take Jodi and Zev "as a reward for what all of you have been through." The trip included roundtrip business class airfare for four to South Africa and a first class private safari for four in Kenya and Tanzania, East Africa. The safari was being organized by Abercrombie and Kent (A&K)—an upscale tour company.

I told Mike that the trip sounded wonderful, especially since the money would all go to breast cancer research. In fact, it all seemed to fit together perfectly until I asked him the list price. He told me it was a whopping $86,000. I chuckled and watched the developing fantasy in my mind quickly dissolve like an aspirin dropped into a glass of water. I knew that the people who attended this fundraiser were high rollers from the cruise industry who sometimes overbid the list price. As I told my son, we were in no position to bid on this trip, not even close.

Mike, being the shrewd poker player he is, simply said, "What do you have to lose? It doesn't cost anything to bid." It was hard to argue with his logic, but I feared getting caught up in something we could not afford. I told him we would sleep on it. Ronnie, a former travel agent, did some research and learned that the airfare alone was close to $9,000 per person. In that context, we authorized Mike to bid up to $40,000 for the trip, thinking and half-hoping that it would never happen. Even that number was a big stretch for our budget, especially when all of the extras were added into the mix. Still, something made us just go for it.

Maybe it was all we had been through in Cancerville and the opportunity to do something healing as a family. Maybe the extra push was the knowledge that we'd be contributing to breast cancer research. Maybe it was what I said about priorities and taking better care of us—perhaps it was all of the above. In any case, we gave Mike permission to bid.

The Seed Takes Root

Mike called the next night while at the event and excitedly said, "We got the trip!" I said, "Really, it went for forty grand?" feeling both happy and worried. He said, "Nope," baiting me in his inimitable style. I said, "I told you not to go any higher." "I didn't," he said. "We got it for $26,000!"

With this information, I breathed a sigh of relief as our budget could handle that amount. It was expensive but doable for us. I realized that it was all meant to be. *Bashert* is the Yiddish expression for that type of experience. From that moment on, we began to call it our "trip of a lifetime." As it turned out, it was, in every possible way.

We called Jodi and Zev, who were unaware of any of this, and told them of our good fortune. We presented the trip to them as an early wedding gift (no pressure), if and whenever they decided to marry. As it turned out, Zev was already planning on asking Jodi to marry him; he had even begun looking for a ring. That romantic engaging moment took place in Napa Valley shortly thereafter. Jodi said she didn't want a big wedding and there was some talk of their eloping. Our only condition was that we be present. No specific plans ever materialized before our trip to Africa.

The Beanstalk Starts to Grow Taller

We arrived in Franschhoek, South Africa, on New Year's Eve at about 11:15 p.m. just as 2009 was coming into view there. Since 2005, we had welcomed every New Year as a further step away from Cancerville.

As Jodi, Zev, Ronnie, and I began to enjoy our time in Africa together, Sloan-Kettering and our experiences there seemed very far away, not only geographically but also emotionally. It became clear that Mike's idea had been nothing less than brilliant. At some point early in our trip, Jodi and Zev, with perhaps a little prompting from Ronnie (again, no pressure), decided that they wanted to get married in East Africa. They called Duncan, our contact person from A&K, who had planned our safari. He said he would see what he could arrange, and Jodi and Zev eagerly awaited his call.

Each time we arrived at a new lodge in Kenya and Tanzania, Jodi and Zev would excitedly inquire as to a plan, but no one had heard a word about it. Calls to Duncan were met with voice-mail or immediate disconnects, as cell service in East Africa has quite a few gaps. Thus, suspense lingered in the air, but we were all so distracted by the amazing sights of being in the wild that the uncertainty about the potential wedding wasn't an irritant to our trip. I think we all quietly adopted a *bashert* attitude. Cancerville teaches patience and tolerance for ambiguity better than any other place I have ever been. If it was meant to be, it would happen.

The Beanstalk Starts to Sway

With only two nights left on our trip, we arrived at the Ngorongoro Crater Lodge where we all simultaneously had the same thought. This magnificent place with an absolutely gorgeous and glorious view overlooking the crater would be an idyllic setting for a wedding. It would be a scene out of a very special movie. We held our breath as Jodi asked, "Have you heard anything about our wedding?" "No Ma'am," came the brief reply, "but I will check into it." The odds of this wedding happening seemed to be approaching zero, but we decided to wait and see. Cancerville taught us not to pay too much attention to the odds, one way or the other.

That night before dinner, the answer finally arrived. The wedding was scheduled for tomorrow. It was set to take place at four o'clock, our last day on safari. "Oh, by the way," we were told, "it will be at the Maasai Village. You will all be dressed in traditional clothing, and the whole tribe will participate." We looked at each other in shocked amazement and excitement. This was due in part to it really happening and in part to where it would be held. Zev broke the tension by saying to Jodi, "Don't worry honey, it will be like Halloween." I couldn't help but silently remember that Halloween-like feeling I had on that fateful day at Sloan-Kettering when I was struggling to deal with what was going on in the OR. This plan for Jodi and Zev's costumed wedding sounded like a whole lot more fun; no tricky treatments this time around!

Climbing the Beanstalk Together

At the wedding, something out of *National Geographic*, Jodi looked like a beautiful tribal princess while the rest of us looked like mere trick-or-treaters. The ceremony itself involved both Jodi and Zev being adopted by tribal parents whose job it was to convince the chief to allow and bless the marriage. Thus, Jodi may be one of the few people adopted twice in her life.

The ceremony took place in the native language of the Maasai, with an English-speaking translator provided. To honor our Jewish tradition, we bought and brought along a Maasai blanket attached to spears to serve as the *chuppah* (canopy) that was held up by four people from the tribe. We also brought an expensive crystal glass wrapped in a linen napkin (please don't report this to the lodge), which Zev stepped on repeatedly and finally broke at the conclusion of the ceremony, much to the confusion of the tribe. Our Muslim driver and guide, Shofino, brought one with him, too, just in case we forgot to bring one. I had explained our custom of breaking a glass to him the day before. His remembering and caring showed the potential for us to all live together peacefully.

They Really Raised the Bar

On the way back from the village to the lodge, we were driven to a special area where a bar overlooking the crater was set up by the hotel just for us. It was oh so much better than the BYOB one in the men's room of Sloan-Kettering. I didn't need a drink at that moment as I was on a natural high. Notwithstanding, I had one anyway to toast the bride and groom. Tradition!

When we returned to the lodge, the staff of fifteen or so Tanzanians was waiting outside to sing and dance with us, which added to the magic of the moment. Then, we spontaneously organized a *hora,* a traditional Jewish dance, only a short distance away from a giant buffalo that decided to join in on the merriment. No, the buffalo didn't dance, nor did his size keep us from celebrating.

The entire staff joined us in this traditional dance and the party was officially on. It was a long time coming, but here it was. It was a YES, tears of joy moment in every way! I could write many more pages about this trip and my daughter's magical fairy tale wedding, but I don't have to. You can see the video, professionally prepared by Zev's video company, Milk and Honey Productions, by going to www.cancerville.com. I assure you it is worth your time. I hope it will help you to start picturing happier and more wholesome images for your own family.

The Seed Takes Root Once Again

Once married, Jodi and Zev very much wanted to have a child, as neither had previously experienced parenthood. Post-chemo, Jodi was told the odds of her being able to conceive a child were not high, especially since she still had five years on Tamoxifin before they could try. Unfortunately, strong chemo can age female reproductive organs by many years. Nonetheless, they went for a miracle, and tried very hard to conceive, hoping and praying their love would be the magic potion—and it was!

Our beautiful granddaughter was born a week before Thanksgiving 2012. As Bernie Siegel, M.D., would say the angels assisted, and the interesting thing is that he has me agreeing with him. We were truly blessed and all are doing just fine— poo, poo, poo. Look what Ronnie has me doing! Between them both I'm not the same person, and that is a really good thing.

We undeniably went from the outhouse of Cancerville, to the penthouse of life in Tanzania amid the Maasai, to the pinnacle when Jodi and Zev's daughter was born. We've been truly blessed and we feel grateful every single day.

In Sum

Never in our wildest imaginations, while we were in the thick of Cancerville, did my family ever conceive of such a healing trip to Africa or our daughter's marriage to Zev in Tanzania among the Maasai tribe. Nor did we ever conceive that Jodi and Zev would be able to conceive this marvelous and miraculous little girl.

Life, as we have all learned, is unpredictable, not just in terribly scary and sad ways, but also in happy ways. For now, please try to see that there can be "happily ever after" times after such unhappy times in Cancerville. My family went from the bleak darkness of Cancerville to the heart of darkness, as Africa has been called, where the sunny blue skies with swirling white clouds looked like a bright and beautiful work of art. And then, a bright and beautiful work of art joined our family.

Assume and believe in some form or other that sunny skies lie on your family's horizon as well. Know that life is full of surprises and *bashert* moments of excitement and joy. Try to look beyond this Cancerville moment and see a much more positive future. It is my heartfelt hope that your loved one can also enjoy warm and positive experiences to salve his or her wounds from Cancerville. Toward that goal, I sincerely wish you well!

A Closing Letter of Caring for Family and Friends ("Heart and Soul Givers") with a Loved One in Cancerville

Dear Family and Friends,

We have been walking together for a while now. You have come to know a great deal about me, while I have not had the opportunity to get to know you. Such is the nature of book communication. Feel free to email me to let me know how things are going with you and your loved one. Your feedback about this book is welcome as well.

I am hopeful your loved one's situation has gone well. I am sincerely sad and sorry if it has not. My goal was to write a clear, supportive, and elegant book about a confusing, overwhelming, and inelegant place. I have tried my best to guide you through this difficult land I call Cancerville. I hope you were able to feel my hand of support reaching out across the miles. I also hope, at least at times, that you were able to replace your frowns and those of your loved one, with smiles. I am very hopeful that you learned some things about yourself and others that apply to life in general, as well as to Cancerville.

I believe that how you let Cancerville shape you is ultimately within your control. You have the power to process your experience as you choose. You can't change what happened in Cancerville and all that you and your loved one have gone through and may continue to go through. You can, however, deal with it in a way that frees you rather than causes you to be a perpetual prisoner.

If your power has been weakened by the journey or the outcome, there are many resources available to help you regain your strength and be able to rebound soon. These include counselors, support groups, spiritual guides, family and friends, websites, books, and anything else that might be helpful to you. In addition to the above, sometimes just a getaway to a spa or other relaxing place helps to clear your mind and recharge worn and depleted batteries of body, mind, and spirit.

Cancerville has already taken so much from you, even if the outcome was successful, and even more if it wasn't. Try your hardest not to let it suck you dry and take away your energy and zest for living. If you must, do battle to reclaim yourself—you are worth it! Even though Cancerville sucks, life, in my opinion, does not.

As I have said, one of the many lessons you learn in Cancerville is that you never know what's coming around the corner. Life is unpredictable and we are all vulnerable to unanticipated happenings that can be positive or negative. In that context, we need to live our lives fully. We need to treat ourselves kindly, and we need to eventually bounce back resiliently from the trauma of Cancerville.

It will take you some time to neutralize the newly acquired cess from Cancerville, but you can do it; I am optimistic that you will. I leave you with one of the very best prayers I have ever encountered. It works for all areas of life, including Cancerville, and for all religions as well:

THE SERENITY PRAYER

God, grant me the serenity to accept the things
I cannot change,
Courage to change the things I can,
And wisdom to know the difference.

I sincerely hope that this book and your own life experiences have helped you find that important wisdom. It is not always easy to know that, but Cancerville does make it a little clearer.

Obviously, I cannot conclude by saying it has been a pleasure to go through Cancerville with you. There is no pleasure in being there. However, I am honored that you allowed me to walk by your side and take and talk you through its rough terrain.

I now slowly and gently withdraw my hand and leave you to go the rest of the way on your own, strengthened from our time together. Here is a fist bump coming at you to acknowledge the strength, courage, and dignity you displayed. Of course, you can always visit me online, read weekly posts on our Facebook page, or return to this book and grasp my hand whenever you might need to feel that symbolic but strong support. It will always be there for you.

I want to leave you with an image I observed on Thanksgiving Day 2011. The family was all here, which is always special. I wandered out to the backyard to water my new red impatiens plants. Jodi and Zev were near the canal, fun-fishing for bass. They were goofing around, teasing and laughing about who was the better fisherperson. Actually, Jodi often is, much to Zev's chagrin. I stopped and took in that tranquil and happy scene. I breathed in deeply and let it out very slowly. I let that joyful moment wash all over my Cancerville cess for a while. These are the simple times for which I feel so grateful!

I had the thought that, like plants and flowers, people need the emotional equivalent of sunshine, water, fertilizer, and weeding. We also need positive images to replace those that are not so pretty. We need to focus on the now so we can get rid of, or at least lessen, the harsh times of the then. My family and I have much for which to be thankful, all things considered. I sincerely hope you do, too, and wish you and your loved ones the very best in all respects and good health from now on.

I dubbed this writing my *mitzvah* (good deed) project. I hope it has touched and helped you in the way I had envisioned. The lovely thing about good deeds is that they come back at us in all kinds of unanticipated ways. Please try to do a *mitzvah* every day and enjoy the multiple dividends that they offer. If nothing else, they will fill your pride bank and, frankly, that is payday enough for me, and I hope for you as well.

God Bless all those who have ever been to Cancerville in the past, those who are there now, and those who will be entering it soon or in the future. God Bless the researchers, doctors, nurses, and medical teams all over the world. God Bless all of us who deserve to be among the blessed. With these blessings, I choose to hope, pray, and believe that you and your loved one will be survivors of this experience.

I sincerely thank you for reading my book. I hope it helped you—and that it was the "home run" I strived to hit!

Your Cancerville friend for life,

Bill

REFERENCES

1. Mukherjee, Siddhartha. *The Emperor of all Maladies: A Biography of Cancer*. Scribner Book Company: New York, 2010.

2. Woznick, Leigh and Goodheart, Carol. *Living With Childhood Cancer*. APA: Washington, D.C. 2002.

3. Siegel, Bernie. *Love, Medicine and Miracles*. Perennial Library: New York, 1988.

4. Brinker, Nancy. *Promise Me: How a Sister's Love Launched the Global Movement to End Breast Cancer*. Random House: New York, 2010.

5. Seligman, Martin. *Learned Optimism*. Pocket Books: New York, 1990.

6. Armstrong, Lance. *It's Not About the Bike*. Berkley Publishing Group: New York, 2001.

7. Siegel, Bernie. *How to Live Between Office Visits*. Harper Collins: New York, 1994.

8. Cousins, Norman. *Anatomy of an Illness as Perceived by the Patient*. Bantam: Toronto, 1981.

9. Penzer, William. *Getting Back Up From an Emotional Down.* Esperance Publishing: Ft. Lauderdale, 1989.

10. Rubin, Theodore. *Compassion and Self-Hate: An Alternative to Despair*. Simon and Shuster: New York, 1998.

11. Byrne, Rhonda. *The Secret*. Simon and Schuster: New York, 2006.

12. Peale, Norman Vincent. *The Power of Positive Thinking*. Simon and Shuster: New York, 2003.

13. Ellis, Albert and Harper, Robert. *A Guide to Rational Living*. Wilshire Book Company: California, 1997.

14. Seligman, Martin. *Flourish: A Visionary New Understanding of Happiness and Well-Being*. Simon and Schuster: New York, 2011.

15. Kreamer, Ann. *It's Always Personal: Emotions in the New Work Place.* Random House: New York, 2011.

16. Kushner, Harold. *When Bad Things Happen to Good People*. Avon: New York, 1981.

17. Goodheart, Annette. *Laughter Therapy*. Less Stress Press: California, 1994.

18. Provine, Robert. *Laughter: A Scientific Investigation*. Viking Penquin: New York, 2000.

19. Klein, Allen. *The Healing Power of Humor.* Tarcher: California, 1989.

20. Gray, John. *Men are From Mars Women are From Venus*. HarperCollins: New York, 2004

21. Kubler-Ross, Elizabeth. *On Death and Dying*. Taylor & Francis: London, 1969.

22. Kroningsberg, Ruth. *The Truth About Grief.* Simon and Schuster: New York, 2011.

23. Becker, Ernest. *The Denial of Death*. Simon and Schuster: New York, 1973.

24. Nouwen, Henri. *Turn My Mourning into Dancing.* Thomas Nelson: Tennessee, 2001.